Vet at the End of the Earth

Vet at the End of the Earth

Adventures with Animals in the South Atlantic

Jonathan Hollins

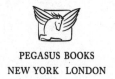

PEGASUS BOOKS

NEW YORK LONDON

VET AT THE END OF THE EARTH

Pegasus Books, Ltd.
148 West 37th Street, 13th Floor
New York, NY 10018

Copyright © 2024 by Jonathan Hollins

First Pegasus Books cloth edition November 2024

ISBN: 978-1-63936-742-9

10 9 8 7 6 5 4 3 2 1

Printed in the United States of America
Distributed by Simon & Schuster
www.pegasusbooks.com

To Teeny, for her staunch friendship; to brother Nick, for being there; and to the islanders of the remote South Atlantic Overseas Territories, British citizens of an indomitable strain who have brought colour and light – and no end of inspiring challenges – to my calling.

And not to forget my hairy family – Che, loyal springer, and Doogs, regal moggy – for their entertaining antics, unconditional companionship and flawless honesty.

Animals represent the best of us. They never lie.
Even to a vet.

Contents

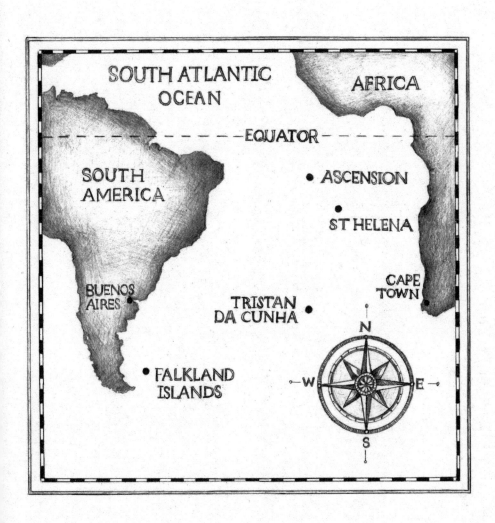

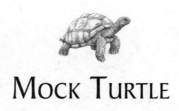

Mock Turtle

IN MEMORIAM TESTUDINIS

ONE of the two oldest and most respectable inhabitants of St. Helena has we regret to state been lost to us, leaving a solitary relict to bemoan its fate. We refer to the decease of one of the bicentennarian pair of tortoises whose existence has been connected to Plantation House during the past sixty years at least. It is enough to make anyone moralize to reflect what changes these two reptiles have witnessed during their almost fabulous lifetime ...

The venerable reptile was deserving of some respect and it is to be hoped that at all events its shell, and skeleton, will be preserved in all due honour. As to its flesh we shudder to relate, *horribile dictu*, it was converted into <u>real</u> turtle soup! A fact.

St Helena Guardian, 20 Sept 1877,
St Helena Island, South Atlantic Ocean

DEATH OF AN IMMORTAL

The Great Interrupter, both friend and foe, jerked me to attention: the office telephone, ringing frantically like a spoiled child.

Most vets develop a loathing of the phone through years of duties and lives interrupted during antisocial hours. This, at

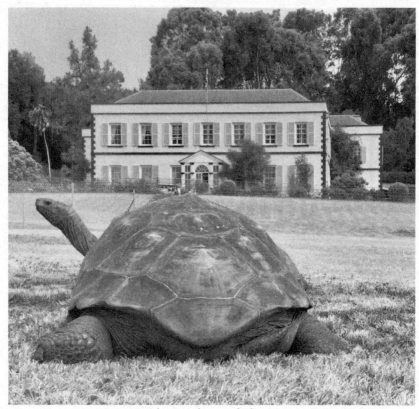

Jonathan in front of Plantation House © Tina Lucy

least, was simply an overcast Monday morning. I dropped what I was doing and grabbed the uninspiring beige receiver.

'Is that the vet?' An American voice with a southern drawl.

'Speaking. What can I do for you?'

'I'm going to ruin your week.'

Oh great. 'OK. What's up?'

'Your big old buddy's dead.'

'I beg your pardon?'

'Your buddy. Dead. Toast. Shuffled off this mortal coil and all that. I think you'll find he's finally departed this life.'

Cocky. Very cocky. Mondays are never my best days as the weekend tends to leave a legacy of problems. I had a pile of visits to do and a cat with a possible blocked bladder that needed urgent attention. The agriculture offices of St Helena stand at an altitude of 500 metres on the edge of the island's cloud forest, and charming though it may be, it also means regular immersions in dank chilling mist. The dim light seeping through my window was beginning to reflect my worsening mood.

'I'm sorry, but it's a bit early in the day for Monty Python. Who is this, please? And who's dead, what buddy?' I could detect a niggling undertone of glee in the American's voice, which was riling me.

'Hey, keep your hair on. I'm just a member of the public doing you a service and informing you that the big old turtle you guys look after is dead. And,' he added smugly, 'it's Shakespeare, not Monty Python. You're a Brit. You should know that.'

Despite his provocation, my irritation instantly dissolved, to be replaced by a rising tide of doom.

Turtles regularly arrive in the island's waters: Green, Hawksbill, and the occasional vagrant Leatherback. And they sometimes even attempt to land and lay eggs. No one really knows why since, apart from the elevated, wind-blown coral sand beds of the eastern coast, noted by no lesser mortal than Darwin as being of a former age, all the beaches are hostile banks of coarse volcanic stone, and turtles are meant to return to their place of hatching. The only time turtles did haul out and plant clutches of eggs in the gravel of the deceptively or perhaps sardonically and even cruelly named Sandy Bay, most were swamped by a storm, and of the thirty or so rubbery eggs we rescued and set in an incubator at the government poultry unit, only one produced a hatchling. This cute little wriggler we ceremonially released back into the sea, to do battle with the seabirds and predatory fish that treat hatchlings like boiled sweets.

But now, a harrowing truth was dawning. In many languages turtle and tortoise are synonymous, for which I blame the Italians (*tartaruga*). For once, they inexplicably neglected their Roman forebears, who had the profound common sense to distinguish a sea creature (*turtur*) from one that roams the land (*testudo*), as do the animal-loving English. But for turtle – in American English especially – read tortoise. It could only mean one thing. The death of a legendary Titan.

'Oh no!' I said breathlessly. 'You mean Jonathan? The tortoise? Do you mean the tortoise at Plantation?' The Governor's grand, imposing residence.

Jonathan was an Indian Ocean giant tortoise, nearly two centuries old. As the oldest known living land animal in the world (a necessarily pedantic definition since Greenland sharks and corals live longer), he was immortalised in *Guinness World Records*. He had received worldwide attention, been the subject of numerous articles in national daily newspapers, and received more than a million views on YouTube. As a publicity machine for the island's fledgling tourism industry, the hoped-for panacea to her economic woes, he was pure gold. And tourists adored him.

Furthermore, he was the island's icon, beloved of the Saints, a symbol of endurance, resilience and longevity in a mercurial world. He had seen world wars and plagues, monarchs and dictators, nations and even empires come and go. And he'd lived through the waxings and wanings of the island's fortunes, indifferent to it all, content in his paddock, grazing grass and mulling over whatever tortoises care to mull about. He even features on the island's coinage, a neat profile of this huge reptile squeezed into the confines of the tiny five pence piece with JONATHAN THE GIANT TORTOISE in paradoxically minuscule letters arched over his domed shell. It has been a neat double act with our longest-serving monarch, Queen Elizabeth II, on the obverse, who even when she passed at the phenomenal age of ninety-six was a youngster half his age.

For the island, the death of Jonathan would be like the ravens leaving the Tower of London: a portentous omen.

And I, as the island's veterinary surgeon, had the great honour and privilege – and overwhelming responsibility – of caring for him.

'You say tomarto, I say tomayto... Yes, the tortoise at the Governor's spread.' Again, that hint of relish. He knew that he was throwing me a hatchet, and playing a starring role in a momentous island event.

'OK.' Pause. Calm, calm. 'Why? Why... do you think... Jonathan is dead?'

'I'm that jogger, Roger Stokes. Used to work at the American base on Ascension. Sure you've seen me. I jog through Plantation Forest every day. He's spreadeagled in the middle of the Paddock, and he's been like that for two days. No doubt – must be dead.'

'Spreadeagled?' Jonathan was close to 200 kilos in weight, and spreadeagling seemed anathema to the species, let alone anatomically improbable.

'That's what I said. Spreadeagled. All four legs at full stretch and his long neck straight out in front of him and flat to the grass like a fence post. You better get down there, son.' He chuckled softly to himself. 'I don't envy you this one.'

Two days in the same place, and somehow slumped out of his shell. He had to be dead. It was shocking news. All I could manage was a trance-like, 'Thank you. Bye,' as I put down the receiver and dropped into my chair.

Jonathan was nearly 200 years old. It was inevitable he would die sooner rather than later. As with all celebrities, we had even prepared a plan – the brilliantly named Operation

Go-Slow – complete with obituary, formulated with my input by a bright wordsmith and Public Relations Officer, Ian Jones, who had come direct from the higher echelons of Whitehall. But inevitable or not, under every governor I had served I had been given one clear injunction, often delivered with a desperate undertone of pleading: 'Joe... not on my watch.' Unfortunately, it was always and unavoidably *my* watch.

I wrenched myself from my chair, sped down the corridor and grabbed my dependable right-hand man, Ken Henry. He read my face.

'Uh-oh. What's up, Joe?'

'It's Jonathan. I think he's dead.'

'Shit,' he said laconically. There was no better word. Ken usually had the verbal dexterity of an auctioneer and never swore.

'Let's go.'

For every human being on this planet, Jonathan had always existed. But it wasn't just the Saints' huge sense of loss that worried me. I was sad. Jonathan was my friend. I had bonded with this noble hulk of a tortoise.

Tortoises are fascinating beasts. And a veterinary challenge. When your patient's body is encased in half-inch-thick armour plating and chain-mailed over the head and legs, textbook clinical examination goes out of the window. The good news is that I have yet to be savaged by a tortoise. Trampled, yes. Rammed, indeed. Even bitten. But not savaged. And Jonathan was the gentlest of them all.

When I first arrived on St Helena, I examined him in as much detail as was feasible. He was clearly in his last years. He was blind with cataracts, especially his right eye, the lens a conspicuous white blob in his dark pigmented orb. He had no sense of smell. His legs were bony and draped in loose folds of dry reptilian hide. His beak, which should have been a double rim of interlocking, razor-sharp serrations designed for scything grass and shrubbery with ease, was soft, blunt and crumbly. I sat for minutes, hours even, observing his behaviour and that of his four companions, an apprentice in giant-tortoise husbandry, and I saw him biting into dry leaves and soil, tugging hopelessly on long strands of tough, rank grass, and mouthing air for food. I realised he was very, very slowly starving to death. And so, once a week on a Sunday afternoon, I began to feed him by hand like a cherished, ancient uncle in an old people's home, although

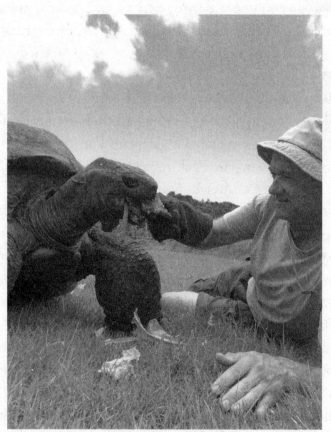

Feeding Jonathan his fruits and vegetables

not with beef soup or porridge but with a boosting tub of fruit and vegetables. The one sense he retained in abundance was his hearing, and he was famed for walking over to the Paddock's tennis court, drawn by the clack-clack of rallies, and standing there transfixed like a fossilised spectator. He even began to recognise my voice. I would collect the tub of fruit and vegetables provided by the Governor's kitchens, don leather welding gloves and softly call his name, at which he would instantly perk up, step forward and start biting at the air. I knew it wasn't a demonstration of primitive reptilian affection, more a Pavlovian response – but I liked to kid myself otherwise.

That this simple act instigated an unexpected miracle of almost biblical proportions and gave this chelonian king a new lease of life, I can't take credit for. I was as astonished as everyone else.

Aficionados will tell you that the feeding of fruit and vegetables to these mighty grazers of roughage should only be done in moderation, or risk metabolic mayhem. For Jonathan, though, it proved his elixir. His beak regrew its finely honed edge, he grazed better, put on weight and became more active. In short, he rejuvenated. His centuries of wear and tear had been leading him down the sticky path to oblivion, but somehow we'd turned him back. It wasn't just calories he had been short of, but those vital drivers of our marvellous and insanely complicated organic processes: vitamins, minerals and trace elements. He was now braced, I hoped, to face his third century of existence.

My affection for him, that innate, empathic link between man and beast, grew and grew. It had become my absurd ambition to make him outlive us all, to keep him going long after I had laid down my scalpel and hung up my stethoscope. But that ambition suddenly looked bleak.

There are a growing number of scientific papers that delve into the genomes of giant tortoises, unravelling the great mysteries of life, because within those magical helices of base pairs lie many micro-secrets with momentous implications. Pet owners know on some level that their dog undergoes the same ageing process in ten or fifteen years as they do in seventy or eighty, yet the simple deduction that follows often eludes them: something has its feet on the brake and the accelerator.

Giant tortoises are rigged to survive, blessed with enzymes to stall the oxidation and ruinous misbehaviour of damaged controller genes known as the methylome, thus preventing or hampering cancer, and to delay the unravelling of the telomeres – the ends of chromosomes that are like the aiglets on the tips of a shoelace. These multiple obstacles to ageing are the key to something approaching quasi-immortality. In fact, some authorities claim that giant tortoises don't really die from old age, at least not in the way we tend to. They simply wear out. It's a bit like a used and treadless tyre; what's left is perfectly intact, there's just not enough of it to function properly. Like Jonathan, before his weekly feast.

At the request of researchers at the Vanderbilt University Medical Center in good ole Nashville, Tennessee, I had lost fingernails retrieving Jonathan's DNA, my leather-gloved left hand acting as an unhappy wedge in his powerful beak while I frantically swabbed his tongue. The United States Air Force Base Commander on our less-isolated sister island of Ascension personally couriered the samples to Patrick Air Force Base in Florida when he went on his Christmas leave, no doubt gaining a raucous anecdote over post-prandial bourbon and coffee about how he'd shipped tortoise saliva across the Atlantic. Then an excited scientist drove 700 miles to collect

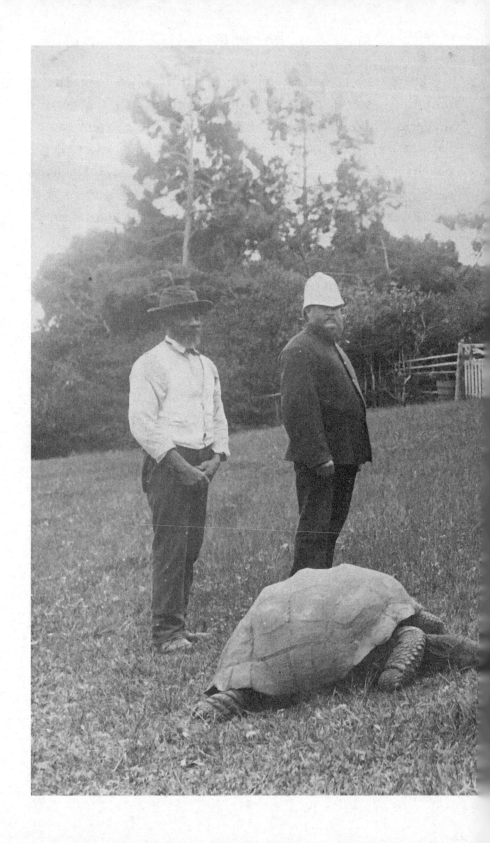

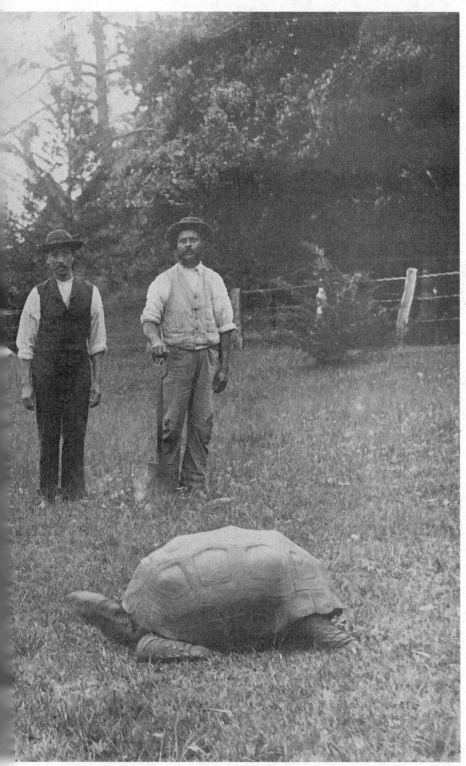

Jonathan (left) in the grounds of Plantation House in the late 1800s them. It was Jonathan's contribution to humankind's long battle against cancer, and the researchers have since successfully unravelled both his genome and methylome and probed their arcane mysteries. Their excitement is almost palpable. Scientific papers are in the offing.

Then there was the other extraordinary fact about Jonathan. His de-extinction.

In the days of ambling square-riggers when mariners relied for their meals on salt beef and ship's biscuit, quite often semi-decayed with a juicy garnish of maggots and weevils, giant tortoises provided a welcome taste of fresh meat in an otherwise bleak and unappetising diet. They were herdable, stackable, didn't require food or water for long periods, and – greatly to their detriment – utterly delicious. It doesn't pay to be utterly delicious, and the world's giant tortoises were all but eaten out of existence. Several species were indeed classified as extinct, until in the late 1990s Dr Justin Gerlach at the Nature Protection Trust of Seychelles had a lightbulb moment.

If they were transported all around the world in the holds of ships, and often gifted in novel acts of diplomacy, then, given their astounding longevity, perhaps some species were not so extinct after all. A deep trawl through the world's collections restored two species from the eternally dead: the Seychelles and the Arnold's. Dr Gerlach sent me a comparison table to distinguish the commonest giant, the Aldabra, endemic to the second largest atoll in the world where 100,000 still roam the mangrove swamps and beaches, from the Seychelles giant. I crawled under and over Jonathan, measuring curved lengths, straight lengths, circumferences, heights, suture lines, scutes and notches, jotting them down with a pencil into a mud-smeared table. Looking over the results, there was no doubt about it: Jonathan was a de-extincted Seychelles giant, a phenomenally rare survivor.

True, the days when naturalists would frantically run about with nets and guns, spot a specimen, kill it, preserve it by drying, gluing and stuffing, measure up all its distinguishing characteristics, call it a species and add it to a reference collection, have been substituted by DNA. DNA rips away ambiguity. It deciphers the biological palimpsest and reveals the hidden text. And it turned out that the Seychelles giant is a subspecies: *Aldabrachelys gigantea hololissa*. Good enough for me.

We could confidently say Jonathan was a de-extincted quasi-immortal, the reptilian equivalent of super powers. But now, it seemed, his bout with immortality was finally over. With furrowed brows and heavy hearts, Ken and I hurried over to Plantation House, fearing the worst.

LYING IN STATE

Plantation House, built by the East India Company in the late 1700s and now home to the Governor of St Helena, Ascension and Tristan da Cunha, is a gorgeous pistachio-green Georgian confection of sash windows and high-ceilinged rooms under steep slate roofs. The huge ornate wooden porch stands on a rampart of broad, foot-hollowed limestone steps, flanked by two bulbous trypots used as planters, and the whole edifice is surrounded by the colourful, well-tended flowerbeds and ancient specimen trees of a sprawling historic garden with stupendous views far out across the Atlantic.

Thick, wrought iron railings pierced by two latched metal gates delineate the house from a steep bank, the equivalent of a ha-ha, that drops onto a levelled field. This is the Paddock, home to the island's small collection of Indian Ocean giant tortoises.

A set of double railings across the bottom of the Paddock creates the tortoise corridor, which is designed not to guide the tortoises in their daily perambulations, but to channel visitors. It is a viewing path that – once they've had their fill of tortoises – steers them down into the allotments below, and thence into the black heart of Plantation Forest to be spooked by the eerily sited Butcher's Grave, the headstone carved with skull and cleaver.

I pulled up the Land Rover in front of Plantation House with a crunch of gravel and looked down into the Paddock. A thin, dissipated sunlight had broken through the chilly murk, illuminating the grass with shades of pastel green. Out in the open in front of the tortoise corridor lay Jonathan, in a wholly unnatural and unlikely posture – spreadeagled, indeed. I had never seen him like this; besides which, the tortoises always took themselves off into the bushes at night and he had apparently been lying there for two days.

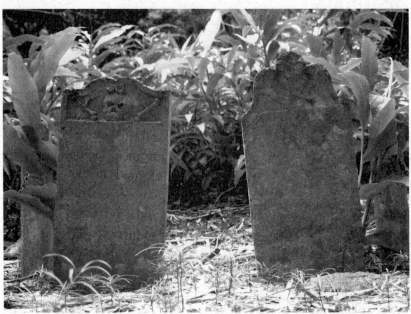

Butcher's Grave in Plantation Forest

'Ken, we're screwed.' A leaden sense of loss was engulfing me. For all my checks, I must have missed something. If only I could seize time by the fetlock and turn it back.

'That's a dead tortoise, Joe.'

'Yup. There's no good dwelling on it. Let's go and see the damage. Then we have to scramble the team for Operation Go-Slow.'

Unlatching the gate, I walked down into the Paddock and somewhat unwillingly approached the stationary, domed figure. Jonathan's neck, evolved for reaching high into shrubbery, had always struck me as snake-like, generously long. I never could understand where he stowed it when he pulled his head into his shell. Alarmingly, its full, almost freakish dimensions were now on display, stretched out flat on the ground, along with all four of his stout legs splayed out like the pillars of a collapsed temple.

I squatted on my haunches a few feet away and contemplated his armoured, angular, greenish-black head, every scale of which I knew so well. His eyes were closed, streaks of rheum wetting his cheeks. It was a forlorn spectacle.

'Strange though,' I pondered aloud, 'I always thought they'd die with their eyes open.' A flicker of hope rose in my heart. 'Wait a minute...'

I prodded his long leathery neck. His eyes shot open as he jerked his head in the air. If there was an expression to be read, it was most definitely, 'What the hell...?' After all, would you poke your great-great-grandfather while he was taking a recuperative nap?

I fell backwards onto the grass and laughed the marginally insane, high-pitched laugh of the greatly relieved. Ken clutched his head in surprise.

'Oh Jonathan! You bloody great fraud.' I gently hugged his long sinewy neck, something he adored as he stole the heat from my mammalian flesh, and he relaxed its length along my forearm.

Yes, of course, it was clear now.

Jonathan was sunbathing.

Here was something I had failed to glean in my self-taught apprenticeship with giant tortoises. This was reptilian thermo-regulatory behaviour. They are poikilotherms: cold-blooded creatures. The weather had been damp and nippy. The tortoise's carapace is a thickly insulated wall of keratin, bonded into the flesh and bone beneath. It is effective at capturing the warmth for the coolness of the night, but equally effective at blocking the intense heat of a tropical sun during the day. When the sun fails day after day, as it so often does during the brief St Helenian winter on the fringes of the cloud forest, then the shell's occupant must seize every opportunity to absorb even the slightest warmth of filtered sunlight. This is best achieved by exposing the largest surface area of skin possible to those beneficial rays. Spreadeagling, in fact. Cold blood out; warmer blood back in. Core temperature raised; metabolism supported. Another night survived.

Thankfully, this majestically long life wasn't yet over. Operation Go-Slow could remain on file.

And the American jogger could stuff his Shakespearian quotes – appropriately – where the sun very rarely shines.

GENESIS

The story of how I came to have the immense privilege – and impending catastrophe – of caretaking the oldest known living land animal in the world – the story of how I came to be the senior vet in this remote location – stemmed from a chance one-month locum, many years earlier, in the subantarctic regions of the South Atlantic. On, in fact, another British Overseas Territory, and a thriving member of the island family: the Falkland Islands.

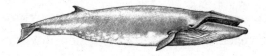

Rite of Passage

The desire to fly is an idea handed down to us by our ancestors who, in their gruelling travels across trackless lands in prehistoric times, looked enviously on the birds soaring freely through space, at full speed, above all obstacles, on the infinite highway of the air.

Wilbur Wright

CARCASS ISLAND, WEST FALKLAND, SOUTH ATLANTIC OCEAN

'Whoaaa!' roared Captain Tom Chater over his shoulder. 'That was close.' We had almost been shot out of the sky by a ground-burst of chunky, feathered projectiles.

Tom's instinct had been unerring; he yanked down the yoke and gunned the revs, throwing the pitch of the Islander aircraft from a shallow descent into a steep tilted climb, all within the fraction of a second. Pure muscle memory. I glanced across at my companion. Shona's face had the numbed look of one who has stepped over the edge, purged of all emotion by the narcotic of excess. It had turned to a pastel shade of lime.

'Bloody geese!' Tom exclaimed from in front. He was one of the pilots with FIGAS, the Falkland Island Government Air Service, and a more adept bunch of sky jockeys would be hard to find. On top of that, the short-take-off Britten-Norman Islander plane was highly manoeuvrable, the right tool for the job. The

Falklands cover an area the size of Wales, an archipelago strewn with islands, each outlying settlement dependent on a grass or dirt airstrip, some of them as tight, curved and knobbly as a whale's back. And the weather is notoriously mercurial: 'four seasons in one day' as the islanders often say. Only the capital, Stanley, and the imposing military base at Mount Pleasant have solid, all-weather runways. Every week the phenomenally able FIGAS pilots string together all the remote settlements and inhabited islands, carrying passengers and provisions, and constantly honing and stretching their skills against meteorological extremes. They are motivated by the knowledge that they allow the islands to thrive, and indeed in the case of medical emergencies, to survive. My admiration for them was unlimited.

'Don't worry,' I shouted in Shona's ear, reassuringly. 'I had a friend who worked for Rolls Royce in Bristol, and they used to fire frozen chickens into jet engines just to test them. No problem.' The fact that those engines were turbines was beside the point.

'Would have made a helluva mess of my props,' bellowed Tom jovially, levelling out the aircraft as he made a lie of my small crumb of intended comfort.

Shona gave me a withering look, now in no doubt that a solid bird strike would have resulted in instant goose liver pâté and propeller blades like wilted flowers.

Tom was nestled in his pilot's headphones and concentrating on the instrument panel, quite unaware of any passenger anxiety in the seats behind him. With one aborted landing he was now circling for a second attempt, staring out through the rain-smeared windshield to decipher the antics of the windsock on Carcass Island's only strip of level ground.

Our projectiles had been upland geese. Upland geese had become emblematic of the Falkland Islands ever since the

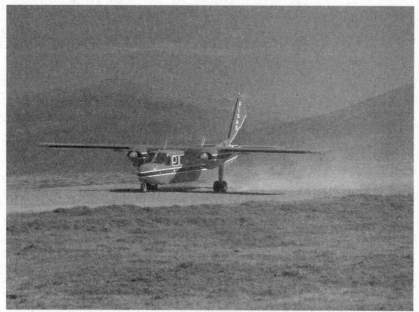

A FIGAS Islander aircraft coming into land

Argentinians used the Upland Goose Hotel in Stanley as their invasion HQ. The geese – and the ubiquitous sheep – had an opportunistic fondness for the lush, short-cropped sward of the grass airstrip, and normally the farmer, whose task it was to prepare and man the strip, would shoo them away. This gaggle, however, had been well concealed, hunkered down in the peat against the incessantly foul weather, and had been panicked into flight by the overhead roar of the plane's engines at the most critical moment of landing.

THE DEVIL WITHIN

Shona and I were returning at the end of a mission on West Falkland. The weather had been vicious: thick swirling mists, punchy squalls and horizontal sleet and rain, with visibility just farmyard deep. West Falkland is the more sparsely populated of the two main islands that lie back-to-back like unidentical twins, but in many respects the more handsome. 'West is best' is the common refrain of its very scattered 'Westers', and I had to admit I was a convert. Although it was a close contest. I was already in thrall to the whole archipelago's beautifully interwoven land- and seascapes: its soft-hued hills, dark blue waters and bright white beaches fringed with chocolate banks of giant kelp.

But on West Falkland the rainfall is generally less, the hills greener and more rounded, the topography altogether smoother and kinder than the harsh, jutting, quartzite ridges of the east. More prosaically, the island is simply an interesting shape, with lots of intriguing attenuated peninsulas, long, deep inlets and fragmented offshore islets.

It has no real hub that equates to Stanley, no large military presence like Mount Pleasant, and the neat farming settle- ments are widely dispersed among the bays, creeks and coves of its wildly convoluted coastline. Interior settlements are few. Like all the Falklands, communication has been reliant on the sea, with shearing sheds backing onto quays and jetties for shipping out the bulky bales of wool. Only relatively recently have dirt roads been pushed into these rural fastnesses, connecting them to each other through the valleys and ranges of the interior, and punching a small hole in their long-held geographical solitude.

I had freshly returned to the Falklands after a previous one-month locum visit, and this mission was my initiation. Vic Epstein, Senior Veterinary Officer at the Department of Agriculture and my new boss, had called Shona and me into his office with a plan to unravel a Houdini act by a notorious parasite.

Shona Strange was the Biosecurity Officer, biosecurity being a gutful of a word that is now second nature to me. It's hard to define perfectly, but in essence biosecurity is a system erected by a nation to protect the environment, agriculture and population from invasive pests and diseases. This particular pest was hydatid.

Hydatid is to parasitology what the movie *Alien* is to nightmares. It certainly isn't dinner talk.

A humble tapeworm of just a few millimetres in length known to science as *Echinococcus granulosus*, it nonetheless has big ambitions. The normal life cycle is simple. The sheep, the definitive host, harbours a tapeworm cyst; the dog, the intermediate host, scavenges a sheep carcass out in the fields, and picks up and develops the seemingly innocuous little tapeworm, in turn pumping out thousands of eggs onto the pasture grazed by sheep. The dog infects the sheep, the sheep infects the dog, and so on, ad infinitum, in a two-host cycle generated through long and close association. And just to ensure the dog is infected, nature knows that there's nothing a dog likes more than to take a pungent souvenir of its sumptuous feast by rolling in the rotting carcass, then licking its coat for dessert.

Unfortunately, it is all too easy for humans to stumble into this life cycle and become an accidental host. The infected dog partakes of its lavatory, licks its anus, grooms its coat, we stroke and pat the dog, pick that annoying raspberry pip out from between our molars, ingest a lovely faecal egg, the egg hatches and migrates, finds a comfortable organ and sets up a factory.

There is no more insidious enemy than the devil within. Over a leisurely five to ten years a cyst develops, incubating what is in effect a hive complete with budding brood capsules, and slowly expanding until it is a sizeable balloon containing up to four million tapeworm heads. A city of clones. Each one is a minute sphere with an inverted crown of claws ready to deploy like grappling hooks. Yes, fiction is benign compared to the horrors of reality. I told you it wasn't dinner talk.

Back in the day, many a Falklander bore a long scar where a cyst had been surgically removed. Some still do. It's a fiddly and challenging dissection with an inherent danger of puncturing the cyst and releasing the swarm into the abdomen. Our over-arching goal was to eliminate this detestable parasite altogether, and we were almost there. New Zealand, Iceland and Tasmania had succeeded, but it had taken decades. All the same, with only 700 dogs in all the Falkland Islands, consigning hydatid to history should have been child's play. The recipe is simple: worm all the dogs, break the life cycle, and deny hydatid an existence. Yet the abattoir proved otherwise. Stanley has a large EU-approved export abattoir, at the time processing some 30,000 sheep a year, the perfect monitoring unit for hydatid, and despite our triple-pronged attack, five bulging hydatid cysts had somehow slipped through the net. Not many, but enough to niggle.

Vic Epstein was a dry and laconic Australian, one-time professor at a university and hugely knowledgeable. I had worked my locum placement under a different boss, Steve Pointing, who was so collaborative and relaxed that we had bonded easily and enjoyed a vibrant and humorous working relationship. So far, I was still getting to grips with Vic's blunt mannerisms and the great void between our cultures.

'Next week,' declared Vic, 'I want you to go a-dog-worming.' He paused for effect.

'Dog worming?' Needs must. My job is full of seedy and un-glamorous tasks.

His mouth flickered with internal amusement. He slid a kidney dish across his desk. A pretty, golden globe wobbled in its silvered depths. 'Yup. I want you to go out West with Shona and do a little sleuthing. This bloody thing...' he jabbed his index finger at the hydatid cyst, '...should be gone. Do some gentle probing. See what you can find out. And see if they know how to worm their bloody dogs.'

Shona, slight of build but hardy, was the daughter of one of the earliest and most successful ecowarriors of the region, Ian Strange. Ian had fought against powerful sealing concerns and later established a wildlife reserve on the southern half of New Island. Since then, the island has been turned into a conservation trust, fostering scientific research and both supporting and improving wildlife habitats – a refuge in perpetuity.

So Shona was a true island child, brought up by a tireless polymath in the cradle of the sea. She was steeped in island life, and as such proved to be a most excellent and entertaining travelling companion. She was also perfectly reared for her role of Biosecurity Officer.

For the two days before we flew, a biting gale laden with snow and hail drove hard through the islands. But on the third day, the day of our flight, the clouds parted and the sun poured forth its dazzling light. The bright-red Islander aircraft flew from Stanley across the heart of East Falkland, weaving through the spine of Wickham Heights and out across the Sound to the West.

It was astounding, my first true experience of the islands from the sky. The hills and mountains were swathed in all their winter glory, mantled in white and marbled by the grey, boulder-packed 'stone runs'. The paths and animal tracks were sharp and delineated like a topographical threadwork of bloodless veins. The Falkland Sound – which splits East and West as a diagonal gash – was dark and still, and beyond stood the eastern coast of West Falkland, a sheer, straight bulwark of mountain pierced by a narrow ravine: the entrance to Port Howard.

The approach is nothing less than thrilling. Beyond the entrance, concealed at first but then slowly revealing itself, lies a magnificent harbour: an inundated valley some eight miles long, forked at the northern end where it lifts into the hills. Here, a sprinkle of buildings embraces a quay, and a few small boats lie at anchor in the shallows. Port Howard and the nearby farms of Bold Cove and Many Branch, with their white-walled, green-roofed dwellings surrounded by a patchwork of bitumen-black clapperboard stock sheds, sheep yards and gorse-hedged fields, form one of the most attractively located and well-maintained settlements on the islands.

It also has one of the bumpiest landing strips, a camel-humped sheep paddock that doubles as an occasional racecourse and was, to top it all, now covered in snow and ice. The best level ground near Port Howard probably lies at the bottom of the harbour.

The Islander bounced like a rubber ball, slewed from side to side, and skidded to a halt. The pilot, as cool and unruffled as the harbour waters below, taxied the nimble plane to a shed where a Land Rover waited, hitched to a fire trailer. A small hand-painted sign tacked to a post proclaimed, tongue firmly in cheek: 'Port Howard Airport'. The pilot stilled the props, walked round the tail, and unloaded our bags onto the snow. Dog worming or not, this felt like living.

We collected the government Rover from a field two miles away, crunching it through the crust of snow and up over a fence ramp. A pair of crested caracaras, majestic, red-faced birds with stern raptor eyes and black toupeed heads, clung to the fenceposts like finials and watched us with stony disdain, splendid against the snowy backdrop. There is no asphalt in West Falkland. It is as if John McAdam never had a good idea. Shona turned the vehicle onto the main track and launched us into our mission.

We arced west around the Hornby Mountains, leaving the peak of Muffler Jack in the rear-view mirror, and headed out along one of the many fingers of coast. On the rear seat, my bag sat bulging with wormers, medicines, syringes and various other

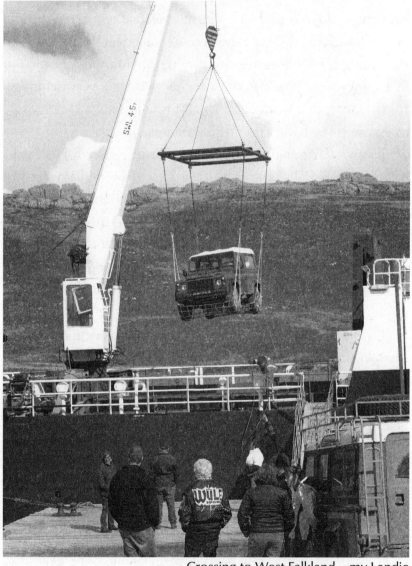

Crossing to West Falkland – my Landie
being offloaded at Port Howard

assorted veterinary paraphernalia for the inevitable and dreaded 'While you're here...'

Crooked Inlet, our first port of call, had an uncanny resemblance to a Cornish fishing harbour, with a tight creek walled in by high cliffs. It made me feel at home. Possibly it was the handful of old, colonial kit buildings perched on the steep shore or the low-roofed shearing shed crouching down by the water; or it may simply have been the sun playing on Hummock Island out in King George Bay. But the clincher was the overwhelmingly friendly reception from Danny and his wife, which I soon came to realise is the hallmark of these islands.

Danny's farm had the feel of a well-run concern. His cattle, beautiful Red Polls, ambushed the Land Rover like a herd of homesick children and would have happily climbed in the back for a lift down to the house. Likewise, when Danny released his dogs from their kennels, they bounced and cavorted enthusiastically around us, and came into the old tack room when called by name to take their wormers not out of fear, but out of a desire to please their master.

Danny's wife insisted that we consume a pot of tea and a mound of cookies before we did a shred more work. We pulled off our boots in the porch and went into the snug warmth of the kitchen. The kitchen table stood in a broad window at the front of the house. Danny gestured to the unparalleled view that spread before us: the creek, the bay, the offshore islands. 'You're unlucky today,' he said apologetically. 'We've had a pod of whales in all summer, and you can stand on the cliffs and look down their blowholes.'

I gawped at him. What I would have given to look down a whale's blowhole and admire the plume of its spout.

'Oh, don't worry, it'll happen soon enough,' he predicted with confidence. 'Plenty of whales about.'

The day wore on and we made our way round the farms in the north of the island: Dunbar, Shallow Harbour, Mainpoint, Boundary, Peaks. Part of my remit was to check out the kennels and the dogs' general welfare. I had to restrain and recalibrate my soft UK sentiments. These were not house dogs, spoiled and pampered at any expense; they were tools of the trade. They had to earn their keep or they became a burden. Nevertheless, they were entitled to certain minimum standards of care. The Hydatid Eradication (Dogs) Order, my legal truncheon for worst case welfare scenarios, stipulated that all dogs had to be confined when not in use, to prevent them following their noses to a nicely brewing sheep carcass or the farmer's offal pit. It was a law that could, with poor management, create a welfare situation, so it was even more important that kennelling was of an acceptable standard. It meant that while I was gently quizzing and advising the farmer on offal disposal and slaughter technique, I was also squinting at the kennels.

No one likes a government inspector nosing around their property. It is intrusive. It smacks of certain negative impli-cations, such as distrust and suspicion of wrongdoing. The trick is to enthuse the farmer, to make it all as conversational and interesting as possible, preferably fuelled by a large mug of tea and a slice of homemade cake. After all, this was also an investi-gation. There was a riddle to solve: the Houdini act of an unholy and tenacious parasite. Hydatid was known and hated by all, and farmers are in touch with their animals and know their environment. They are worth listening to, and their suggestions and observations are usually on the mark.

What about blue buzzers? Yes, I could tell them, flies are known to transmit eggs over several hectares. Feral cats? This question came up frequently. Only lions, I would reply truthfully, lightening the mood. How about the turkey buzzards that regurgitated pellets around the settlements? Apparently, with typical canine good taste, dogs found these pellets particularly morish and wolfed them down like treats. An astute local observation. I made a note. And foxes? Aha. They could indeed play a pivotal role in the affair.

It was known that foxes could also act as a host, supplanting the part of the dog and existing outside any control measures. There are no foxes on the main islands, but the Patagonian fox, or grey fox, *Dusicyon griseus*, had been introduced to seven off-shore islands – Staats, Weddell, Beaver, River, Chain, Split and Tea – in the 1930s in a doomed attempt to establish a fur trade.

The introduction of the fox to these islands has been an ecological disaster. Many of the ground-nesting birds, such as the tussock bird, Cobb's wren, military starling and Falkland pipit, already jeopardised by the feral cat and the European rat, have been decimated. Furthermore, in places the fox can account for some 30 per cent of lambing losses, even though it has adapted well to scavenging on the shoreline and feeding off insects such as camel crickets. Beautiful though the animal is, it is not indigenous to the Falklands, and the local wildlife pays the price. That, by the way, is a classic example of a breach in biosecurity.

Several of these fox islands had sold substantial numbers of sheep onto the main islands, and they were strong contenders for creating a hydatid loophole. I added it to my list.

CANINE CHOREOGRAPHY

By the end of the second day, Shona and I were cold, mud-splattered and stinking of dog matter. The floor heater in the Rover was cooking my boots and I was gradually being asphyxiated by wafts of unspeakable intensity. It was late and very dark, but we had one more task in hand: to visit a pair of pet dogs at Little Chartres on our way to our beds in Fox Bay.

Little Chartres stands on the banks of the crystal-clear River Chartres, which tumbles down from the foothills of Mount Moody through a low-walled gorge. It is one of the islands' most bounteous trout rivers.

I jumped out to open a gate and paused to take it all in. Somewhere below, the water splashed and gurgled on its tumultuous journey to the sea. Above me, a pure, moonless night, unmarred by streetlamps or vapour trails. I had forgotten how inexplicably crammed the southern sky is. The peerless black of space was pierced by innumerable points of fiercely scintillating light, shorn in two by the spiralling arm of the Milky Way, a dense and discernible smoke of stars.

I was falling under the spell of the Falkland Islands, where nature holds sway in all its raw beauty. At that moment, staring into deepest space, lit by a billion worlds with the river swirling by, I could even forgive myself for smelling of dog shit.

Jim and Leslie, the owners of Little Chartres, had tastefully extended and renovated the house and were in the process of doing up an old shepherd's shanty further along the valley. With rooms to spare, an abundance of trout, and a shanty that could offer the authentic island experience, they had flung themselves into tourism as a primary source of income.

We sat in their kitchen nursing the inevitable mugs of tea in front of a revitalising stove. Leslie placed a hefty cauldron of thick mutton stew on the table and filled two generous bowls. The dogs, recently assaulted with worming tablets, shed their disgust and watched our spoons ply back and forth with envious eyes. The stew was tasty, fortifying and very, very filling.

'A little more?' Leslie's ladle hung poised ready to scoop.

'Well, yes, perhaps just a little, thank you...' She filled my bowl for a second time. I was sure I heard a dog sigh. I shovelled another gluttonous quantity of stewed mutton down my gullet, then laid the spoon to rest, replete and swollen bellied.

'Some more?'

I made a frantic gesture with my hand. More, and I would explode. 'No, no... really... thanks. It was totally delicious.'

'A cake?' Leslie was nudging a tantalising plate of home-baked cakes towards me. The chocolate gleamed, moist and intense. It was quite unfair.

'Maybe just one...'

'I forgot to tell you,' piped up Shona later, as we were driving off on the last leg of our journey. 'There was a bit of a mix-up. Leslie said, "Do you want some dinner?" so I said yes. But I haven't told Deirdre.'

'Deirdre?'

'Yes, Deirdre – where we're staying tonight.' Then she added as an afterthought, 'She's an extremely good cook.'

An hour later we were in Fox Bay Village, once more in the bosom of Falklands hospitality. Deirdre loved to feed people. She rubbed her hands together gleefully and walked over to a heated trolley in the corner of the room. It was groaning under the weight of food. She lifted the lids, filling the room with billows of fragrant steam.

'I thought yoose could be a mite peckish after all that dog worming. Help yourselves.' She stood aside with a flourish. It was a feast, a banquet, enough for a conquering army. My stomach groaned.

A platter of honeyed chicken legs stacked into a pyramid; rows of Pyrex bowls brimming with roast and boiled potatoes, carrots, cauliflower in white sauce; bacon and stuffing rolls; and a small bucket of thick onion gravy. Finally, the *coup de grâce*: fudge cake and cream. Two full Falkland dinners, copious and intensely calorific. I went to bed that night so heavily ballasted that I could barely climb the stairs.

The following day was the fourth we would spend worming dogs, and it was getting harder to remain enthusiastic. When I stepped out onto the village green, fully booted, triple fleeced, with padded trousers and ski gloves, and the hat was mockingly torn from my head by a squall, I knew we were going to have a beast of it that day. Even HMS *Liverpool*, our stalwart island guardian, was visible offshore taking shelter in the lee of the Heads. The weather had closed in, the wind was building to beyond gale force, and the dirt roads were deteriorating into potholed mudbaths.

We ventured out onto the south-west peninsula through attractive, undulating hills topped by bizarrely shaped tors. The whole scenic peninsula dangles from the body of West Falkland by a slender, two-mile neck of land, just like its larger counterpart Lafonia on East Falkland. It would only take a small rise in sea level to split the two main islands into four.

At the end of the track lay the picturesque settlement of Port Stephens, and down a side-branch the farm and old sealing station of Albemarle run by the dynamic Leon Berntsen. This was a brand-new dirt road, opening up an interior previously only seen by shepherds and sheep. The road to Port Edgar, on the other hand, was still incomplete. It had five miles to go.

The incumbent farmer at Port Edgar, Tex, was helpful beyond the call of duty. 'Go to the end of the new road where there's a big government grader,' he said, 'and wait there. I'll come out on the bike with the dogs.' He was going to combine our visit with shifting a mob of sheep and save us hours of hacking on foot across miles of waterlogged peat.

We waited and we waited, but no Tex. He was known to be a reliable, efficient, hard-working farmer and he would not let us down. The weather was worsening again, and I began to get a little concerned. While Shona manoeuvred the Rover to find a signal for the 2-metre radio, I climbed up onto a nearby ridge to scan the hills and valleys.

'Look out for any unusual movements of sheep,' shouted Shona. 'He'll not be far behind.' The landscape was speckled with sheep as far as the eye could see, heads down, grazing into the wind. When they lift their heads in unison, or bunch and flow, there is sure to be a cause nearby.

After a few minutes Shona came up to join me. 'I got hold of his wife,' she shouted into the wind, 'and apparently he left some time ago. I hope he's all right.'

'Well, if he doesn't appear soon we should go looking for him,' I replied.

'There!' She pointed, arm outstretched. A multitude of sheep had appeared on the opposite hillcrest, rimming the skyline in a milling band of white. For a moment nothing happened, then a lithe, dark shape shot out from the rear of the flock, arced wide around the flank, and dropped to the ground motionless like a small, obsidian sphinx. There was no mistaking a collie at work.

The orchestration of animals that followed was mesmerising, the epitome of flawless shepherding. Suddenly there were five dogs fanning out strategically around a torrent of sheep as the flock poured down into the valley, each one darting then dropping, darting then dropping, tucking in the edges of the flock, forestalling breakaways, and nudging the head of the flow.

They seemed guided by an invisible hand, each thoroughly aware of the others and working together as a pack. It is really the coordinated hunt, readily seen in the painted dogs of the Serengeti, and collies possess the instinct in droves. The shepherd harnesses and disciplines these instincts for his own means. It is predator on prey, but without the kill.

The flock pooled in the valley bottom, held by the cordon of dogs, and a man on an ag bike crested the hilltop, silhouetted against the backdrop of scudding cloud. He pulled up abruptly and surveyed the scene, then raised a hand in welcome.

'Isn't that something?' marvelled Shona.

'Pure canine poetry in motion,' I agreed, thoroughly entertained. I felt like bursting into applause.

Tex ran his bike into the valley and rescued a couple of ewes mired in a ditch. We climbed down from our craggy ridge to meet him. In the shelter of the blade on the big government grader, we shook hands and talked hydatid, while the dogs held the flock in check.

Yellow oilskins covered Tex from head to toe, but the mud had sought out every gap, flecking his face and clinging to his rain-soaked moustache. He was quietly spoken and full of good suggestions, and my pen flew across the pad as I jotted them down. He dug into his pocket for some tablets and, calling each dog in turn, relieved them of their station, wormed them, and sent them back. It was a perfect performance.

The days were closing in on midwinter and the light began to fail at four. By the early evening we were on our last call, a small farm at the end of a long track. As we approached the gate, a figure could be seen in a glistening waterproof, braced against the wind and swinging a flashlight. We braked to a stop. It was Susan McBrae, grim-faced, waiting for our arrival. Rain dripped from her nose and chin, and the gusts tore at her hood. 'You the vet?' she asked bluntly. The accent was strongly Scottish.

'Yes. Sorry, have you been waiting long?' I sensed some unhappiness, and mistakenly thought it was directed at me.

'Got your gear with you?' Not a trace of a smile.

'My gear? Yes – some. What do you want doing?' The storm was in full swing, sucking and hammering at the farm buildings and rocking the Land Rover like a toy. It was neither the time nor the weather for wrestling with stock. Suddenly I realised she was on the verge of tears.

'I've got two auld sheepdogs need puttin' doon. They're in the shearing shed.'

The raised shearing stand in a shearing shed is very much like a stage, and usually as well lit. The two old dogs, litter-mate sisters, sat happily on the planking being petted by their master and mistress while I prepared my equipment: syringes of barbiturate, fresh sharp needles, hair scissors, stethoscope, and spirit swabs – not for sterility but to clarify the vein. Despite the weather, her husband had his Land Rover outside with a mattock and spade in the back to complete the job. It was better that way.

Euthanasia is a sorrowful affair. I think if I ever lose that twinge of sadness my time as a vet should be done. Whatever the reason, I am still terminating a life. But the reason is always sound; as a vet bound by the ethics of my profession, it cannot be otherwise. Mainly it is debilitation, often cancer, occasionally severe injury, sometimes organ failure, and from time to time intolerable aggression.

In this case the dogs were beyond working age. The chance of rehoming retired sheepdogs in the Falklands is precisely zero, and feeding the extra mouths is a luxury most farms can't afford. Farmers often take them out for a final walk and shoot them. It seems hard, but then so is farming, and it is quick, thorough and humane. It is also unpleasantly messy, so our visit offered a more palatable alternative.

Usually with gentle holding, reassuring words and a swift purposeful injection technique, the dog is more or less unaware of anything happening, and the deed is done. The drug is a concentrated barbiturate anaesthetic and completely painless. In fact, I often tell people, quite truthfully, it is going out on a high.

Susan cuddled each dog in turn and raised their veins, a brave act which put the dogs at their ease and saved me from struggling with a tourniquet. I quietly sent them both away. The two sisters lay side by side on the shearing stand with the unnatural stillness that comes only with death. I made a routine check of their hearts and nodded.

'Thank you,' she whispered. 'Thank you very much. Please – come inside for a beer. I think we could all do with one.' And with that, through her evident sorrow, she gave me a glorious, radiant smile.

SKY JOCKEY

Dawn on day five broke over a bay in turmoil. Tufts of spume tore from the wave crests as they curled and frothed belligerently in the driving wind. The dogs of West Falkland had all been thoroughly wormed and we were meant to fly back to Stanley for a weekend of detoxing, but the prospect of a long soak in a hot bath and a glass or two of Chilean red was looking decidedly slim. A dank, depressing murk was rolling over the landscape, driven in impenetrable banks by the westerly gale. The visibility was so poor that – almost unheard of for those

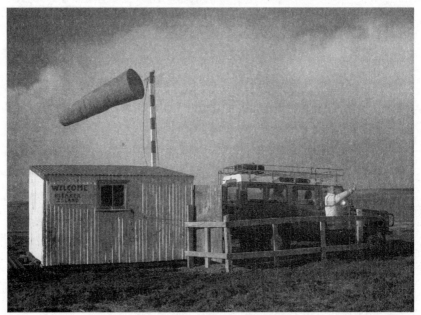

A typical Falklands landing strip at Bleaker Island

unshakeable pilots – FIGAS had already had two no-fly days in a row.

We were sitting having breakfast with our hosts, Deirdre and Gavin, when the 2-metre radio crackled into life. By 2007 mobile phone technology had reached the environs of Stanley, but no further. The radio appeared to require fluency in another language. 'Lizbethvoyscuminin. Canyulendahandwitharopesova?'

For Gavin, though, comprehension was immediate. 'Yup,' he replied succinctly. Then, rising for the door, he said, 'The *Elizabeth Boye*'s coming in. It's a bit tricky. They need a hand with the ropes.' The MV *Elizabeth Boye* was one of the supply vessels that plied between Chile and the islands.

Shona and I shot each other a calculating glance, and in silent agreement jumped to our feet.

All Fox Bay had to offer this long merchant vessel was a short jetty ending in a nub of a landing stage. Bringing in a vessel side-on against a lee shore in a gale is contrary to the physics of staying afloat, but this captain was a gamer, known to consider Fox Bay his most exciting port of call because he enjoyed the challenge of a tricky landfall. He dropped a bow anchor in the bay, let out cable to lower the vessel downwind, and kept the stern seaward with a side thruster. Masterfully done.

Half the village had turned out, gloved and overalled, to moor the ship and unload the cargo. Falklanders are not ones to sit idly by. I found myself braced around a bollard taking up a tug-of-war position and hauling on a stern warp with a pair of farmers. My job description had changed yet again.

The ship was successfully tamed and made fast, and the settlement resupplied.

Another day, another probable no-fly; the weather was just as awful. Shona made a series of phone calls to farmers near potential landing strips for updates on the local weather and relayed them to FIGAS. FIGAS was unsure. The upshot was that if a plane did get through, it would most likely land at Fox Bay because it had one of the best strips. Captain Tom Chater, also a gamer perhaps, decided to roll the dice.

We stood in a small, disconsolate group by the landing strip's fire shed, eyes and ears straining for the possible approach of the plane, but the long protective arm of the coastal ridge was buried in a leaden bank of low cloud. We were pessimistic. Surely Tom had turned back.

But there it was: at first the distant wavering buzz of a mosquito, then the more insistent drone of a bee. And with a dramatic flash of her crimson fuselage the Islander burst through the base of the cloud like an avenging angel.

Tom taxied the aircraft to a halt and quickly loaded the passengers. He was calm, cool and collected, but the pressure was on. 'We're a little bit pushed,' he said, doing his instrument check and clicking various switches. 'The weather's closing in again. First stop Carcass, then home to Stanley.'

I have always enjoyed flying. Never more so, in fact, than in a light aircraft where the view is good, and the presence of the pilot and a bank of instrumentation make the experience tangibly real. Unfortunately, poor Shona, despite being an island child with a lifelong dependency on air transport, did not share my enthusiasm. The view wasn't just good, it was shoved in our faces. It was the most exhilarating flight of my life, but for Shona the most torturous.

Carcass Island lies at the outermost edge of the north-west, with the mass of West Falkland and its many intervening ranges inconveniently in the way; also, now, inconveniently concealed. The devilishly low cloud had interred the hilltops and mountains in fluffy but fatal obscurity, leaving only a thin layer of visibility sandwiched over the lowest of the land. It demanded precise visual flying.

Tom snugged the ground, seeming to hop the fence lines and clip the grass, cleaving flocks of panic-stricken sheep in his wake. He flew tight across sand-bound lakes, along slender fingers of creeks, hopped over broad bays until he reached the cliff-bound west coast, then clung to the rim of the very cliffs themselves before leapfrogging the neck of a peninsula. All around, the fog banks heaved, rolled and threatened, at one stage barring our way completely until a thin corridor of clarity peeled open to reveal a valley. It was breathtaking – both figuratively and literally.

In Christmas Harbour, where the Chartres River debouches into the sea, a pack of marauding sea lions were leaping and scything through the water as they gorged themselves on the spawning trout. And as we were skimming over King George

Bay just out from Crooked Inlet, where our tour of the West had begun, Danny laid on a whale sighting.

I was looking straight down into the wind-ruffled waters when the waves beneath suddenly took on a darker hue, a shadow rising from the deep. A huge glossy head parted the sea and an inverted cone of spray shot high towards the aircraft. For a brief delusional moment it looked like it might envelop us, then it collapsed and vanished, and I was staring into the blowhole of a sei whale. Its long domed back rolled on smoothly through the surface as it slid out of sight.

In the excitement I grabbed Shona's arm. Shona was by now in extremis, and she, undoubtedly thinking a propellor had come off, let out a small shriek and banged her head against the window.

And then, to cap it all, we were nearly shot out of the sky by the flurry of upland geese.

At the second attempt, the geese having fled, Tom made a safe landing on Carcass Island. He dropped off the other passengers, did his walk around the craft, plucking and prodding at her structure and making sure the wings were still firmly attached, then gave us a pre-flight brief. 'Well, the weather's closed in and there're just too many mountains in the way,' Tom said matter-of-factly, standing tall in his navy-blue overalls, epaulettes shining. 'So I'm going to show you just what these superb machines are capable of. We're going to jump over everything.'

Shona groaned.

'Not to worry,' he told her confidently. 'It'll be cold, but I might even find you some sunshine.'

He wasn't kidding. We took off and Tom immediately put the plane into a steep, parabolic climb through the enveloping white. We could have been suspended in a chamber of cotton wool. Only the intensifying cold gave away the increase in altitude, until Tom was forced to switch on the heaters. Shona fell silent and her pale face took on the torpor of the nearly dead.

It seemed endless. But with a sudden ripping of the vapours from her wing tips, the little Islander leaped out into luminous sapphire skies, trespassing into the high-altitude territory of her larger cousins. Then, as if following the arc of an arrow, she crossed the two main islands to plunge once again into a blanketing fog and grope for her approach to Stanley Airport.

The fog was tight to the land, blindingly white. Tense moments passed. But just as we thought Tom would be forced to make an instrument landing – luckily, at the one airport where this was even possible – the plane broke through and shot past the comforting black-and-white sentinel of Cape Pembroke lighthouse. Stanley Airport lay directly ahead. Shona slumped in exhausted relief.

'Well? What do you make of the West?' Sarah Bowles, practice manager, veterinary nurse, floor-sweeper, penguin-wrangler and general factotum of the government veterinary service, had come to pick us up. Golden hair, freckled cheeks, sparky and bright, often sharply sarcastic and funny, she was an indispensable and highly capable colleague and would become a close friend. She also knew how to roast the most tender, succulent, herb-encrusted mutton in the southern hemisphere. And she was biased; she was a Wester.

'Bloody wonderful. I've been well and truly initiated into your dark tribal arts,' I gabbled happily, still zinging from the journey.

'West is best!' she affirmed. 'And the flight?'

'Exhilarating...!' I was lost for words. 'Your pilots are incredible.'

'Oh yes,' said Sares with a knowing smirk. She was married to one of them. 'Shona, you OK?'

Shona glowered. 'No!' she growled. 'It was terrifying.'

40

Sares gave her a sympathetic squeeze and, turning to me, set her lips in mock severity. 'Righto. Holiday over. So... what do you know about Patagonian toothfish?'

'Pata what?'

She shook her golden head and tutted. 'Oh dear. I thought so.'

Not much. Not much at all. But I was about to learn in a baptism of fire... and fish.

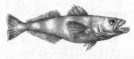

TOOTHFISH

Be fruitful and multiply and fill the earth and subdue it,
and have dominion over the fish in the sea...

The Bible, Genesis 1:28

IRON MAIDENS OF THE DEEP

There is a voracious predator of the southern seas that is more
succulent than salmon, more expensive than tuna, and more
toothy than barracuda: the aptly named Patagonian toothfish.
One of the world's leading authorities on the toothfish stood
before me, waist deep in seawater, looking on paternally and
with admirable nonchalance as fourteen of these oceanic raptors
circled his legs.

Dr Paul Brickle, marine ecologist and toothfish supremo,
had sharpened his own teeth on his PhD, *The parasite ecology of
the Patagonian toothfish*, required reading for other toothologists.
The Patagonian toothfish, and its cousin the Antarctic toothfish, each oozing with an oily antifreeze which gives the flesh its
succulence, are well-established in Antarctic waters and exploited
by all adjacent nations. And more besides. Until recent times it
has been a species much preyed upon by illegal fishing vessels
and is so sought after by epicureans that it has earned itself the
moniker 'white gold'.

Fishing is in the lifeblood of the island economy, and Paul
was a key player in the proficient and tightly run Fisheries

Department, which monitors and controls fish stocks, principally to sustain them for the benefit of future generations. The department is located on a relic of the 1982 Falklands War: FIPASS. A more bizarre complex of offices and laboratories would be hard to imagine.

The Falkland Interim Port and Storage System was one of those permanent temporary solutions to a vexing logistical problem: that the otherwise excellent Stanley Harbour had no deep-water wharf, a prerequisite for cargo handling during post-war development and the construction of military facilities. FIPASS is a floating dock. Fortunately, it was supremely overengineered and has well exceeded its life expectancy. It consists of six giant pontoons chained together three by two. Along one side, echoing, battleship-grey metal warehouses rise from the decking, with converted ship containers welded onto their flat booming roofs like stacks of bricks on a parapet.

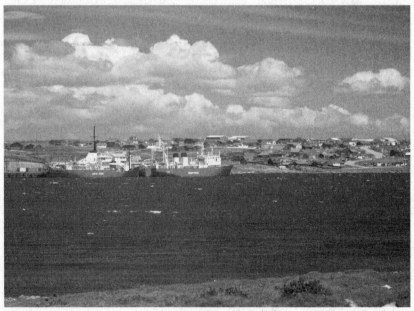

Stanley viewed from across the harbour

Here and there, hole-punched steel steps climb to meet gridded walkways. FIPASS is a monstrous, bobbing village of metal, which oscillates to the thrum of the water, and bangs, grinds and moans to the thrust and pull of the winds and the tides. If the world was made of steel and water – nothing else – this is how it would look. It is anchored off Stanley foreshore and reached by a matching Meccano-set bridge.

The Fisheries Department operates from its own jumble of converted containers, now pierced with windows and doors, and welded together into a disorienting maze of rooms and corridors. The varying slope of all the floors and the subtle, almost subliminal motion of the pontoons give the visitor the distinct feeling of mild inebriation.

Paul had led Vic and me into one of the loftiest chambers of this metal complex where, to our surprise, we found a substantial PVC swimming pool. An oxygenator burbled and gurgled, and a pump swished in fresh seawater from the harbour way below. Paul climbed into a shiny aquamarine drysuit, donned dive boots and gloves, and swung his legs over into the pool while wielding a landing net. He was stockily built, with a useful layer of natural cladding for his diving exploits in achingly cold waters. His round face gave him a boyish, even impish look, but his eyes shone with knowledge and a fierce passion for all things briny.

'They say you have an interest in fish?'

'An interest, yes, but I'm not a marine biologist,' I replied as disarmingly as possible. I didn't want to appear cocky. It is true that I had developed an interest in freshwater fish, both tropical and pond, and this had extended to fish farming after seeing practice in Cumbria with an inspiring fish vet, but to claim I was an expert would be a blatant fib. All the same, a great attraction of the Falkland Islands was that, alongside Vic, I was now involved in one of the most prosperous and diverse fisheries in the world. As the presumptuously named Veterinary Competent Authority, we oversaw a fleet of twenty-one EU-approved, mostly state-of-the-art fishing vessels. As a lover of the briny myself, I relished every fish scale.

'So let me introduce you to *Dissostichus eleginoides*, the Patagonian toothfish.' Paul flicked a switch and the lights in the tank changed from soporific red to daylight yellow. The fish were a slatey grey, tinged with brown, and their long, overshot mouths and huge eyes gave them a slightly gormless expression. Their interlocking scales glittered like chain mail in the bright light. 'Not exactly good lookers, but their flesh is highly prized and mostly exported to the States, a pretty valuable resource. We monitor two main cohorts, one off the Falklands, the other down off South Georgia, and use observers and tagging to make sure that there are no shenanigans and the fisheries remain sustainable. These, though, are mere babies.'

'Babies?' queried Vic. The fish hovering around Paul's boots looked ample to feed a family of six.

'Oh yes. The truly large specimens have mostly been fished out, but I've dealt with individuals that weigh 100 kilos and are seven feet long, and I can tell you that's a mouthful of teeth you wouldn't want to engage with. They could easily encompass a man's head.'

There was an image to fill my nightmares. My scalp tingled and I gave an involuntary shudder. Paul showed us a picture later, shot straight into the maw of one of these monster tooth-fish: a broad, batrachian mouth that opened like a handbag armed with several rows of backward-slanting, knitting-needle teeth running deep into the throat. A piscine paper shredder. No escape from that iron-maiden grip.

'So why do you have baby toothfish bobbing around in a swimming pool on top of a warehouse high above the harbour?' Vic asked drolly. 'It's certainly not for the view.'

'These fish can take fifty years to mature and live down to 3,000 metres below the surface, so they're very hard to study and that makes it extremely difficult for us to estimate remaining biomass. Get it wrong and before you know it, we've fished them out. Every fragment of knowledge that we can glean from open-water and captive studies takes us to a greater understanding of their quirks and needs. In fact, here we're also trying to get them up to sexual maturity to establish if there is any possibility they can be bred and farmed. That would be a total game changer. The trouble with captive studies – which is what this is – is that we can't recreate the proper habitat. And that's probably why we're in trouble. Three dead, and others on their way.'

Which is why Fisheries had called us out.

'You said one fish is unaffected. So what's the story exactly?' Taking a clinical history, even for toothfish, is a vital element of reaching a diagnosis. Everything has a pattern, and vets, like paediatricians, have to be detectives because our patients don't talk. There is always a reason – no matter how tenuous, always an answer – no matter how obscure; but sometimes the reason is unfathomable and the answer is unreachable. The fact, though, that one fish seemed unaffected was already piquing my interest. It was a diagnostic hook of significance.

'We call him Blind Len. You must understand that these are voracious predators. For research purposes we need them intact so we can't longline for them. Instead, we catch them in traps set at depth, then haul them to the surface very very slowly, giving them time to adapt. But they thrash around and injure themselves. Len was the first fish, caught some time ago. The others are recent additions. He beat himself up badly and damaged both his eyes. In fact, he literally lost one of his lenses, hence his name. We nursed him for weeks and he all but died, but then incredibly he turned a corner and adapted to his new environment. Everything healed up, he began to eat, coloured up nicely and put on weight. Now he's pack leader. But he's the only one without lesions. It seems he's in some way immune.'

'He's already been through what they're going through,' I mused. 'A virus? A bacterium? Or is it behavioural? He's tame, the others are still wild, so he's fully habituated. Lack of stress?'

'Maybe. Either that or he's a carrier, a sort of Typhoid Mary. So, you've brought some gear?'

'Not a lot, I'm afraid. But you said they had skin lesions, so I've brought the one and only antibiotic we have for fish, enrofloxacin.'

Paul nodded. 'Ah yes, know it well. And the dose?'

'I've got the dose for koi carp.'

'Koi carp?' Vic raised a cynical eyebrow.

'The vet formulary isn't exactly overendowed with doses for Patagonian toothfish,' I replied, a little caustically.

'It'll do,' Paul cut in swiftly. 'Koi carp it is then.' He brandished his landing net. 'I'll give you the worst one first.' He gently scooped up a fish that was wallowing listlessly on the bottom of the pool and lifted it to the surface.

Vic and I threw each other pessimistic glances. The fish lolled appallingly in the water, shedding scales and strings of mucus against the fabric of the net. There were extensive blemishes around the head and eyes, and swarming, discoloured, patchy lesions which were coalescing along its body. Daubs of red showed where the skin had ulcerated through to the flesh. This was a Lazarus job.

'You know how to inject these?' asked Vic dubiously, watching me draw up a dose in a syringe.

'I reckon so. Avoid the abdominal cavity, inject into the dorsal musculature, and angle the needle up against the lie of the scales.'

He nodded approvingly. 'Go for it, then.'

Paul laid a restraining hand against the fish while I injected the antibiotic, then eased it back out into the depths of the tank. It immediately capsized, wreathed in a cloud of separated scales, then slid to the bottom like a spent torpedo. Its gills were motionless.

'Now look what you've done,' observed Vic drily. 'You've gone and killed it.'

'Looks a bit that way. Or maybe it's just passed out?'

Vic vented a derisive snort. 'Passed out?'

Suddenly, in a moment of miraculous resurrection, the fish darted across the pool, shaking its head from side to side as if to expel a demon, then shot to the surface and struck a support strut with an ominous thonk. All meaningful movement once again ceased and the fish drifted to the bottom, belly up. This time it was certifiably stone dead.

'Nah,' drawled Vic. 'You definitely killed it.'

'Best thing to happen,' said Paul, unfazed. 'Now we can conduct a proper post-mortem and take our samples. Let's treat the rest, then do the business.'

It seems perverse to say I love a post-mortem, but I do. It is a hugely informative procedure. Standard practice with fish and poultry, where numbers are usually vast, is to remove the barely alive and worst affected, euthanise them, then forensically take them apart in pursuit of an answer.

The other toothfish were treated without further fatalities, and we adjourned to the laboratory. We squeezed past piles of squid beaks, fish otoliths, sectioned teeth from beached pilot whales, bottled parasites and other assorted paraphernalia from the watery world, to reach a stainless-steel drainer.

Paul laid out our recently deceased as Vic peeled a scalpel blade from its packet and fashioned a handle from the foil wrapper. Paul slit open the belly and teased out the organs, then drew out a variety of parasites and reeled off their Latin names – a cestode cyst here, a coiled nematode there, and a fluke or two from around the gills – but nothing more than expected from living in the wild. He slid them under the dissecting microscope so that we could see how grotesquely well designed they were. Parasites were his thing.

'Ah, my old friend *Anisakis*.' He held up a small worm coiled like a watch spring. 'Sounds like a lovely lady, but this one can kill you. Really surprisingly common.'

'You're kidding?' I quite like an ingenious parasite myself. 'Why would a fish that lives 3,000 metres below the surface in subantarctic waters carry a worm that can kill a human? We're never going to meet. Slightly beyond my dive range.'

'Accidental host. You forget – the sea is full of mammals. It's not meant for you, it's meant for some hapless seal. Personally, I never eat raw fish unless it's been thoroughly deep frozen. Sashimi is a great way to get infected.' He grinned at my expression. This information was going to alter my menu choices for ever. 'Don't worry, Joe. Deaths are pretty rare. It's more likely just to make you bloody ill.'

Vic was nose down in the fish. 'Guts look unaffected – apart from being empty. Doesn't look systemic.'

He sectioned the lesions: minimal depth. I pulled out the dorsal fin: a loose array of bones held together by the vestiges of a membrane; classic bacterial fin rot, but that could be secondary to a primary illness. I lifted the gill flap, the operculum, and peered inside: perfect. Then I noticed something important: the operculum is lined with skin on both sides; outside, it carried lesions, inside it was flawless.

'Vic, look! The protected areas are unaffected.'

'Aha!' He lifted the neat, semi-circular pectoral fin with the tip of his blade. It was set in the midst of the coalesced lesions. Beneath, exactly outlined, was an identical semi-circle of immaculate, unaffected skin. 'Got it.' Vic rolled the carcass experimentally. The lesions were only on the raised contact areas, and the naturally protected areas were unharmed. We exchanged a triumphant grin.

'They're abrasions,' said Vic to Paul, 'from thrashing about when you caught them. Then they've got infected by some opportunist pathogen.'

'And Blind Len,' I chipped in, 'is calm, so no abrasions. He's no carrier, he's possibly not even immune. He's just habituated and completely chilled.'

'Makes sense,' said Paul. 'And we're pumping in harbour water. It might look clean but then the harbour receives effluent from the town, so they're being exposed to novel primate bacteria. Enrofloxacin covers a whole bunch of nasties.' He looked relieved. 'We might just have done the right thing.'

It was still serious, but at least it wasn't some exotic virus. We took a swab and sent it down to the King Edward Memorial Hospital to be plated up on agar and incubated, no doubt, nestling alongside Joe Bloggs's persistent urinary tract infection.

Back at the Department of Agriculture, an isolated 'L' of single-storey buildings on Bypass Road, which ran along the ridge above Stanley, Sares was busy formatting fishery certificates.

'How were the toothfish?' she asked, looking up.

'Fascinating, Sares. But very sick. I managed to kill one of them.'

'Oh well done. Nothing like establishing a reputation. Start as you mean to go on,' she said sardonically. 'By the way, I've booked you to do an end-of-season transhipment inspection on Saturday, a massive reefer vessel called the *Bukhta Omega*. You're on duty anyway.'

'That's fine. What's a reefer vessel?'

'Basically, a big fat floating freezer. The fishing vessels tranship their catches into her so they can go back out to sea and replenish their holds. She'll be stacked to the nines with *Loligo* squid then she'll be off to Vigo in Spain. Should be interesting. Oh, and she's Russian, by the way.'

'Russian? I don't speak Russian.' Most of the fishing vessels had Spanish-speaking crews, the officers drawn predominantly from the maritime region of Galicia in Spain and crew from Montevideo, the capital of Uruguay. I could usually get by with my hesitant Castellano, gleaned from Latin American travels and cycling in Spain. But Russian...

'You'll cope.'

That evening, wrapped up against the cold drizzle, I meandered along Stanley's waterfront, taking in the atmosphere. Stanley has a dynamic port, and the steep face of the settlement is immersed in maritime activity: the comings and goings of the co-owned Spanish trawlers, the rust-streaked Taiwanese jiggers, the bright-red fishery patrol vessels and the ice-class British Antarctic Survey ships.

I stood in the dark on Victory Green between cannon and Hotchkiss guns, the sea slopping quietly at the foot of the wall, and looked across the broad waist of the harbour to where Wireless Ridge, scene of fierce fighting to reclaim Stanley from the Argentinians, was silhouetted against a murky northern sky. Behind me, the monumental mizzenmast of Brunel's SS *Great Britain*, rescued from nearby Sparrow Cove, reclined on its concrete pedestals, dripping forlornly in the rain.

The juxtaposition of so much diversity enriches life. It was a Friday night, the weather was awful, but I revelled in it all.

EL CAPITÁN'S TABLE

Stanley is blessed with an outer, more capacious anchorage which parallels Stanley Harbour and has ample room for deeper-draft vessels: Port William along with its appendage, Berkeley Sound.

Packed with tonnes of frozen transhipped *Loligo* squid, the reefer vessel *Bukhta Omega* stood out in Berkeley Sound alongside the FV *John Cheek*, awaiting my inspection. As an EU-approved inspectorate, I was mandated to put the competence into the Veterinary Competent Authority.

Essentially, the EU delegates the responsibility of monitoring food quality to vets on site, and it was down to Vic and me to ensure that all fish caught were killed, processed, packaged, labelled, frozen, stored and generally handled in a hygienic, documented and legal fashion, so that quality was maintained and the consumer safeguarded. This meant checking the fishing vessels pre-season, end-of-season, and for every transhipment of fish from one vessel to another. Having spent the summers of my youth fishing for the kitchen of my parents' thirteenth-century inn on the South Devon coast, I was truly in my element.

Modern fishing vessels are multimillion-pound labyrinths of ingenious design woven compactly and efficiently into the strict aquadynamic confines of a steel hull, topped by the all-seeing eye of a bridge pulsing with electronics. Only in this way can fishing in the brutal zone below the Roaring Forties be survived and be made economically viable. But for sheer style upon the High Seas, it's the Spanish who take the *bizcocho*: they bring Spain with them. They are also extremely hospitable.

My very first fishing vessel inspection had been during my one-month locum under the wise, guiding hand of senior vet Steve Pointing. Significantly, our embarkation had clashed with lunchtime, and a Spanish fisherman in port is not to be denied his *almuerzo*. The captain, a typical Galician with seawater for blood, invited us to an *almuerzo de trabajo*, a working lunch.

Steve laughed delightedly. 'That's extremely kind of you,' he said, addressing the captain. 'My colleague and I would be honoured to share lunch with you. But work first, pleasure after.' Steve muttered sideways into my ear: 'Well worth it, Joe.'

Inspection completed, we were shown into the officers' mess. A long table draped in white cloth laden with cutlery, side plates and napkins filled the confined space. Portraits of company fishing vessels were screwed to the wood-panelled wall, and ceiling lights bathed all in a convivial mellow glow. I was immediately transported into an authentic simulacrum of a Spanish restaurant, only nautically themed with sea views and portholes.

We took our seats, the officers in order of seniority, and with elegant poise a waiter swept in, spotlessly dressed in white shirt with requisite black bowtie, black trousers and shiny black shoes. He was balancing a collapsed pagoda of small plates along his arm: a *tapa* of *boquerones*, anchovy fillets in herbs and white wine vinegar, and *mejillones*, mussels in tomato sauce. Plate after copious plate followed, the waiter working almost invisibly, clearing away and replenishing, the whole bellyful of food beautifully anointed with a perfectly warmed bottle or two of Rioja Reserva. Which of course had been uncorked in ample time to allow the wine to breathe and evict, as the waiter said, *los pequeños diablos*: the little devils.

The captain raised his glass. '*Salud!*' he said amicably.

The *Bukhta Omega* would be a different barrel of fish. I had looked her up: a 130-metre Russian freezer vessel built in a Ukrainian shipyard in 1987 and named after Omega Bay in Sebastapol on the Crimean Peninsula. Perhaps we would be offered a shot of vodka and a warming bowl of borscht.

THE BEAUTY AND THE BEAST

It was my first time going solo as an EU Inspector. I wanted to at the very least appear moderately competent. I pored over the checklist and tried to commit it to memory: temperature records, cleaning schedule, disinfectants and degreasers, catch compounds, factory conveyors, tunnel freezers, packaging materials, date stamp, approval number, fishing zone, vessel name, call sign, fish species, total catch, fishing dates, transhipment dates,

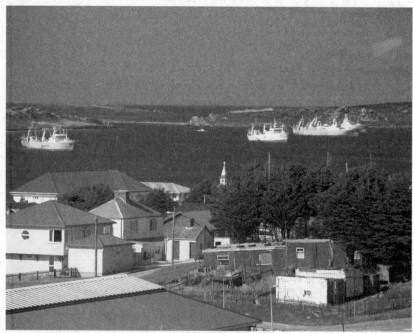

Fishing vessels in Stanley Harbour

water sample, catch sample, bathroom cleanliness, toilet readiness, general unsteadiness... I was nodding off already. I tossed the list aside and set the alarm for an early start.

Saturday dawned bleak and colourless, but abnormally calm. A thick fog clogged the harbour. I parked the Rover by the old East Jetty in the historic heart of the commercial waterfront and walked down to the jetty head, where Stuart Wallace, the owner of the Fortuna fishing company, and his worthy assistant Mike stood ready and waiting.

Stuart was affable. 'You must be Joe.' He stuck out a hand, his shrewd appraising eyes giving me the once-over. 'The launch is late I'm afraid. It's caught up ferrying people to HMS *Liverpool*. Astonishing weather. The harbour's an absolute millpond.' The delay was good; it gave me time to explore. 'I'll leave you in Mike's capable hands,' he added with a barely perceptible nod of approval, and strode away down the jetty.

Alongside the jetty head lay an impressive old lady, the barque *Egeria*. Stanley Harbour is an open-air maritime museum, a treasure trove of wrecks sunk as pier heads or used as storage hulks, potent reminders of the days of sail, when the Panama Canal was still only a concept and all was risked to round Cape Horn against violent prevailing winds.

Remarkably, the *Egeria* is still working. Built in 1859, she received a thrashing trying to weather the Horn on her way from London to Peru with a cargo of cement. Taking on water – and her cargo presumably solidifying into permanent ballast – she crawled back to Stanley where she was condemned and scuttled as a storage hulk.

Half of her still remains. I ran my hands along her fissured wood. Her curvaceous hull towered above me, her sharply countered stern making a shelter for a pontoon on which a seal pup regarded me with doleful black eyes. The surface planking had pulled away in several places to reveal the mastery of her construction, the inner layers of diagonal timbers snugged neatly together and fused to the outer by rows of wooden treenails. Yellow moulds and pale green lichens had colonised the defects and bejewelled the wood with a richness of colour and texture that, even in the dullness of the day, made her look glorious.

The hull had been roofed with sheets of corrugated iron and a crude doorway cut through at the level of the jetty to make a monumental storage shed. Inside, among heaps of coiled warps and tottering stacks of paint pots, the arched oak ribs and thigh-thick deck beams looked as good and as strong as the day they were laid.

The approaching hum of an inboard motor told me that it was time to don the mantle of government inspector and abandon my romantic ponderings on the Age of Sail; beautiful yet deadly.

The fog had thickened into a complete white-out, and the launch chugged through the silent blankness in a sea so surreally static that if it was not for the V-shaped wake rippling out behind us, we could have been motionless with the engine ticking over in neutral. Then, a slight greyness appeared in the heart of the white, took vague form, and focused into the shape of a fishing vessel. She was relatively petite, avocado-hulled, and had a graceful flare to her bow: the FV *John Cheek*.

As we closed in, the glaringly white background behind the *John Cheek* began to dim; a dark, foreboding cliff rising into apparent infinity. A heavily loaded cargo net bulging with cases of squid glided out of the *John Cheek*'s hold and soared vertically into the foggy heavens, vanishing from sight before coming back limp and empty. The gods were obviously laying in stores for a grand fish supper. Somewhere up there, at the end of a very long, rather insubstantial rope ladder, was the *Bukhta Omega*.

First, though, I had the relatively simple task of boarding the *John Cheek*.

My first impression was my abiding one. This was a tightly run ship. I was met at the top of the rope ladder by the Spanish captain, a serious-looking professional seaman with an extremely courteous manner.

'*Buenos días, Capitán.*' I gripped his hand. '*Soy el veterinario del gobierno.*'

'*¡Hablas español!*' He broke into a welcoming smile, ushered me onto the bridge, and settled me down with a sheaf of documents. A *café con leche* slid into view at my elbow. Things were looking up.

Satisfied with the paperwork, I asked to see the hold temperature records and inspect the factory deck – rather charmingly called in Spanish, *el parque de pesca* – the fish park. The first mate led me down along the open trawl deck, stepping over heavy cables and mounds of net, then we descended into the heart of the ship: the engine room.

It was a temple of engineering. Not a trace of oil, a blemish of rust, or a smear of diesel marred the perfection of the shining engines. They were seated centrally on their mountings like idols, serviced by pipes and tubes and an entourage of valves and gauges.

The temperature monitoring device for the freezers was encased, like a Cyclopean eye, on the centre of the bulkhead; a roll of graph paper moved through it at an imperceptibly slow speed beneath a series of styli, leaving an interweaving scrawl of prettily coloured traces. The Chief Engineer handed me a box of old rolls. It was my duty to see that the freezers had not failed during the voyage and spoiled the squid, rendering it unfit to eat. The chances of this occurring were remote because the system employed alarms and back-ups, and the likelihood of the crew covering up such an event was next to nil. Nonetheless, a job is a job. All was in order, and I left the engineers with a tagliatelle-like pile of unravelled temperature graphs, which with typical Spanish good humour they insisted on re-rolling themselves.

'*Todo está muy, muy limpio* – very, very clean,' I said to the First Mate as we mounted the ladder.

'Engineers,' he replied scornfully. 'Much pride in their engines. They love them more than their *madres*.'

Onward we went, wending our convoluted way through the core of the vessel. I peered into the catch pounds for fish scales and slime, the hydraulic hatch poised over my head like a guillotine; I ran my finger under the conveyors for stinky grease; I checked the packaging for correct markings, slid my hand around the hydraulics for leakages, looked into the tunnel freezers for debris. I even checked the toilets had soap and took a water sample to check their tanks for bacteria. The EU has exacting requirements, which on paper may seem pernickety, but in practice mean one can relax and enjoy delicious seafood without fear of a prod in the guts from Neptune's avenging trident. Unless, of course, the restaurant screws it up.

I took out my clipboard and scribbled on the checklist, trying to look as unofficious as possible. '*Está perfecto, Capitán.* You keep a fine ship.'

He gave a gracious nod, eyebrow raised in contentment. 'Of course, *Señor*. I am happy to hear you say it.'

It was time to board the reefer vessel.

Pity the reefer vessel. Unloved and unlovely, it was never meant to be a graceful ship. As long as it is buoyant, stable, large enough to achieve economies of scale, and can move around the world, it has satisfied the purpose of its existence. But this does nothing to confer it with beauty.

Mike called up the launch, and we eyed the daunting steel hull of the *Bukhta Omega*. 'She might have a rope ladder on the port side. Better than sloshing around in the cargo net with a pile of squid.' I was inclined to agree.

The launch edged around the *Bukhta Omega*'s plump and ungainly stern, parting the fog as she went. Sure enough, down the middle of the otherwise featureless metal cliff hung a lank rope ladder, luring us in like a poacher's snare. It vanished into the nothingness, calling for an act of faith that it wasn't a magician's trick and simply tied to a balloon.

'Ahoy there!' a ruddy-faced customs officer who had joined us bellowed up into the ether. 'Hello!' There was an eerie silence. 'Strange. Let's board anyway.' He gave the bottom rung a violent yank. 'Twice,' he said emphatically, 'twice I've had a rope ladder give way when I was halfway up. Some seamen don't know their knots from their arses.' He yanked it again for good measure.

I looked down into the unusually tranquil water, which was only a few degrees above freezing. 'Falling in here would be pretty shocking.'

'Shocking?' he roared. He thumped a stanchion with a grimace. 'A cold dousing and die of hypothermia or strike this and spill your brains like a rotten tomato? As it was, I was left swinging like a bloody pendulum.' Suddenly the soles of his shoes were disappearing past my forehead.

'I wouldn't stand there if I were you.' The pilot, who was steadying the bow against the side of the vessel, threw me one of those 'idiot landsman' looks. 'If he falls, he'll break your neck and leave you in a wheelchair.'

Next went Mike. He was a tall, willowy man with a slight, off-balance tilt to his head who looked as if a gust of wind might topple him over, but he was as nimble as a spider.

Now it was my turn. 'Take it on the top of the rise,' warned the pilot, with slight relish, 'otherwise the launch'll come up and crush your legs. Always three points of contact, or before you know it, you'll be splayed on my deck like a beached jellyfish. And keep your body straight to the hull, or the ladder will fold up and throw you off.'

He could have written a jolly little pamphlet: '20 Ways to be Killed or Maimed by a Rope Ladder'. It was all sound advice that I came to appreciate in future years of boarding vessels in tricky seas. But I couldn't help sensing his morbid anticipation.

The rope ladder didn't betray my lack of experience, and so I failed to entertain the pilot. I made it to the handrail intact where I found Mike peering from left to right in extreme puzzlement.

'It's very peculiar,' he said, 'but there's nobody here.' A slightly bemused kelp gull eyed us from a warp. 'They'll be over the other side,' he continued confidently. We half crossed the deck and peered into the abandoned hold. No one. Even the derrick was deserted, its load half dealt with, cases of frozen squid tumbled from the net. In all directions the deck was lifeless. We decided to tackle the bridge.

The climb to the bridge five decks up was a trial-and-error exploration of doors and corridors, but still we met not one member of the crew. Finally, we popped out into an open expanse, the bridge itself. The bridge is the brain of the ship, normally a lively, exciting space filled with instrumentation, colour and light. This bridge was monochrome, its equipment boxed and panelled in utilitarian grey, its ship-wide view entirely negated by the blanketing fog. It was also completely deserted.

'It's the *Mary Celeste!*' Mike scratched his head. The situation was becoming comical. We had boarded the ship unseen and taken command of the bridge. This was piracy made simple.

And then, quite silently, in this pale grey world, there materialised a pale grey man. I never saw him walk in; I never really even saw him appear. He was just suddenly there. He was tiny in every respect, with a perfectly round, pale grey head, pale grey beady eyes, and pale grey clothes devoid of any rank.

'Er, hel... hello!' I stammered, slightly taken aback by this ghostly apparition.

'Aah!' The edges of his mouth crept out into a crisp horizontal smile. '*Kapitan* this boat,' he announced.

'Captain?' I shook his hand enthusiastically. 'Big ship!' I said stupidly, making expansive gestures. My Russian small talk was extremely limited.

'Big? *Da*, is big.' He shrugged dismissively and puckered his mouth. 'Is only job.'

I felt a twinge of pity. Clearly the poor man was bored. Hanging around in a featureless sound at the bottom of the South Atlantic waiting for vessels to come and deposit their fish was probably not the most inspiring or rewarding way to spend his seafaring days. Nor did it require any of the hunter's skills employed by the other captains.

'Inspector from government,' I continued. 'Temperature fish?'

'*Da, da.*' He was almost animated now. 'I find Chief Engineer. Crew haf break.' And he put his hand to his mouth to indicate taking a drink.

I turned to Mike. 'So that's where they are. Does that mean tea or vodka?'

Mike grinned. 'Knowing the Russians, both I should think.'

The Chief Engineer was a total contrast to the small, grey captain: thick set with a broom-head moustache and wild, bristling eyebrows. He was fresh off his break, and the heavy odour of Balkan tobacco clung to his clothes. His moustache rose on the back of a friendly smile and he beckoned for us to follow.

We descended to deck level and entered a side cabin. Above a rudimentary work bench, a row of oversized dials displayed the temperatures relayed by each and every sensor dispersed throughout the freezer holds. Open beneath the dials was a wide, hardback logbook, its pages drawn into columns with headings in Cyrillic, and every four hours for every probe a meticulously neat hand had pencilled in the noted temperature. They were all in the region of -25°C. No automatic readout here, only a good old-fashioned manual record.

The Chief Engineer turned the pages and ran an oil-engrained finger up and down the columns. 'OK?' he said.

'Perfect!' I turned to Mike. 'It may be labour intensive but it's a thoroughly professional job.'

'It needs to be. There's probably six million pounds' worth of squid on board this vessel.' I looked at him in astonishment. 'A pound a kilo wholesale, and we've stowed six thousand tonnes,' he explained. I wondered how many plates of calamari six thousand tonnes of squid would make and got lost in the calculation. 'But a pound wholesale per kilo... by the time that hits the restaurants...'

'Oh yes. Even with wastage and processing, you could multiply the six million by a factor of ten or fifteen. We're not shelling peas, you know,' he added cheerfully.

The Chief Engineer handed me a pair of gloves. 'Come look. We go down.'

Ladder after ladder we descended deep through the holds into the belly of the ship, our shoes slippery, the gloves preventing our fingers from sticking and ripping on the icy rungs. The Chief Engineer's breath rimed his prodigious moustache with frost, and he took on the appearance of one of Shackleton's finest. Six million pounds' worth of squid was tightly stacked in thousands upon thousands of ten-kilo cases, block upon block, bulkhead to bulkhead. It was mightily impressive.

'You need sample?'

I did. Catches were routinely tested for pesticides and heavy metals, squid having a natural affinity with oceanic cadmium. He pulled out a case and tucked it casually under his arm, apparently indifferent to the -25°C block solidifying his armpit.

'I carry,' he said emphatically, no doubt rightly surmising that I was likely to plummet down three sets of steel ladders and end up as human *calamari*.

At last, my job was done. The Chief Engineer escorted us to the rope ladder. The deck and hold were now abuzz with activity, and the crew, refuelled by whatever beverage it may have been, were hard at work squeezing in the last few boxes. The reefer was crammed to the deck beams.

'We go Spain,' said the Chief Engineer, as I prepared to swing out over the sea onto the rope ladder with my newly gained confidence. 'Ship full.'

'Good voyage!' I took his nutcracker hand. I knew one word of Russian, and this was the moment. '*Dosvidaniya*.'

His moustache bristled with pleasure. He crushed my fingers and pumped them vigorously. '*Dosvidaniya*, friend!' he cried. '*Dosvidaniya!*'

Back on shore, I let myself into the empty offices and walked through the laboratory to the rear of the building. Tucked in a corner at the back stood a large commercial chest freezer labelled 'FISH SAMPLES'. I tugged open the lid and the freezer exhaled a puff of icy steam.

It was neatly divided into two. A laminated notice on the left said: 'TO BE SAMPLED', and on the right: 'SAMPLED'. Suzanne Halfacre, the laboratory technician, had already told me that even though the fish product was generally packed in ten-kilo cases, she needed only a mere fifty grams for the EU testing regime. Once sampled, she moved the rest of the case to the right-hand side of the freezer. 'Help yourself,' she'd said. 'Perk of the job. It only goes to waste otherwise.'

I plonked the block of *Loligo* squid into the left-hand side and, relieved of my hand-numbing burden, went into my office to offload my documents and life jacket. There was a note on my desk from Sares. Ms Efficiency had been in. 'Good news. Call me,' it said, succinctly.

'Sares?'

'How was your Russian?'

'Awful. But everyone was really helpful. And the harbour was bizarre, so still and deadened by the fog.'

'Yes, it's never like this. Anyway, I thought I'd let you know: Paul Brickle called to say that all the toothfish bar one have improved dramatically with the antibiotics. He's delighted, by the way, so they may have you down there again in spite of the fact that you murdered one of his babies! And I put the lab report on your desk. Pseudo something.'

I grabbed the sheet of paper. 'Ah yes. *Pseudomonas aeruginosa*. Well, I'll be damned. It's a common opportunist in both humans and animals, though surely never deep-water fish. It'll be the harbour water. The bacteria gets into wounds and causes havoc. Most antibiotics don't work, so – guess what, Sares – we generally use enrofloxacin. That's the very antibiotic we used.'

'You're a fish doctor already. Even though enrofloxacin was the only one you had for fish anyway – but I won't tell anybody.'

A successful conclusion to an exceptional week. Time for a little celebration. I went back to the freezer and rummaged through the menu on the right-hand side, stacking cases of obscure and unfamiliar Antarctic fish species into a tottering tower: hoki, blue whiting, grenadier, rock cod, even icefish with its strange translucent flesh. But I had my eye on something special, something I had never tried before.

And there it was. I laid my hands on an unusually small, five-kilo case. In bold, blue font on the outside it stated:

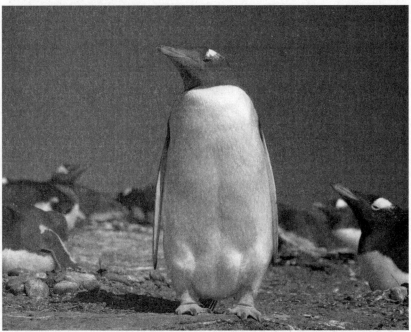

Gentoo penguins at King George Bay, West Falkland

'*Dissostichus eleginoides* – PATAGONIAN TOOTHFISH – Cheeks'. The prime cut of a prime fish. I broke out a generous portion for my supper and laughed inwardly at my self-reward. It felt slightly treacherous to eat my patients, but what the hell...

'Sorry, guys!'

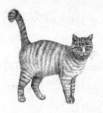

THE TROUBLE
WITH TORNADOS

MSG BEGINS.

HQ LFFI PORT STANLEY. IN PORT STANLEY AT
9 O'CLOCK PM FALKLAND ISLANDS TIME TONIGHT
THE 14 JUNE 1982, MAJOR GENERAL MENENDES
SURRENDERED TO ME ALL THE ARGENTINE ARMED
FORCES IN EAST AND WEST FALKLAND, TOGETHER
WITH THEIR IMPEDIMENTA. ARRANGEMENTS ARE IN
HAND TO ASSEMBLE THE MEN FOR RETURN TO ARGEN-
TINA, TO GATHER IN THEIR ARMS AND EQUIPMENT,
AND TO MARK AND MAKE SAFE THEIR MUNITIONS.
THE FALKLAND ISLANDS ARE ONCE MORE UNDER THE
GOVERNMENT DESIRED BY THEIR INHABITANTS. GOD
SAVE THE QUEEN.

SIGNED JJ MOORE.

MSG ENDS.

Falklands War surrender telex sent by Major General
Jeremy Moore to GCHQ, 14 June 1982

SERGEANT BODDINGTON
The two Royal Air Force officers stood before me in the consulting room, their faces etched with anxiety. Sergeant Boddington sprawled listlessly on the table. It was clear that he was seriously ill.

For sixteen years Sergeant Boddington had patrolled the air traffic control tower at Mount Pleasant Airport. Sixteen years in which he had achieved rank.

Established not long after the Argentinian invasion in 1982 and lying thirty-three miles down a treacherous dirt road from Stanley, MPA is an integral part of MPC, the Mount Pleasant Complex, which is home to some 2,000 service personnel. The irrigated lawns and golf course, with estates of low, green-roofed chalets nestling around a sprawling core of similarly green warehouses, sheds and munitions depots, create an eco-friendly pool of colour against the tawny backdrop of the hills. Its slumbering, peaceful appearance is a deliberate deception, belied by the four-metre-high razor-wire perimeter fence, the no-nonsense airstrip and the squadron of deadly Tornado jets brooding inside their hangars. It is a military deterrent and, if necessary, a deadly killing machine.

The Tepid War with Argentina had become particularly frosty of late, with the seizure of fishing boats and the loud clatter of diplomatic sabres being hurled down distant marble corridors, and MPC's presence was like that of a tough but amiable bodyguard: slightly distasteful yet ultimately reassuring. As air traffic controllers came and went – as all service personnel came and went – Sergeant Boddington stayed, a rock in a sea of change, there through all hours to welcome the shifts and give them the benefit of his world-weary wisdom. There for every landing and take-off, for every crisis, false alarm or emergency, to soothe frayed nerves by his omnipresence, with a simple calming stroke of his luxuriant pelt.

Sergeant Boddington, as he was named in his official light-blue RAF folder, was a handsomely marked, sixteen-year-old, neutered male, ginger tabby cat.

Generally known as Boddy, he served as regimental mascot. Despite his illness, his condition was excellent for his age: thick boned and broad headed, with a full face and a fine spread of whiskers. There was no doubt that Boddy had lived the life of Riley and been fed the very best. It was obvious too from his demeanour that he had been much loved and handled.

But now he stared dully at the wall. His coat, intense marmalade stripes of the thick-cut Olde English variety, was oily and clumped, his mouth pale and tacky, and his eyes rheumy with mucus. I tented his skin; it sank slowly and glutinously back into place. He was dangerously dehydrated.

And then there was a distinctive smell, the smell of rotting fish, of urinals, of an unclean stable: the smell of ammonia. More precisely, of urea, ammonia's vehicle.

Our mammalian bodies are full of toxins, many of which are safely harnessed facilitators in the functioning of our cellular organelles – the nano-engines of our metabolism. Others are the noxious by-products of our day-to-day existence, the effluent of our biochemistry. Among the latter is ammonia, the foul jetsam of protein metabolism, neatly emasculated by the liver which packages it up as urea and sends it to the kidneys for expulsion. Not for nothing is urine called urine. And if the kidneys, those marvellous, complex mini laboratories, are compromised, then urea accumulates in the body and ammonia is liberated to wield its weaponry. Together, they poison the system, make the patient feel nauseous and anorexic, and can even ulcerate the gut. Boddy didn't just smell of urea, he reeked of it. It was the odour of corrupted tissues. It was the odour of death.

I glanced up at the two uniformed airmen. Matt, who was evidently the senior, looked seriously concerned. No doubt my facial expression spoke volumes.

'Is it bad?' he asked tentatively.

'Yes, I'm afraid so. See his coat? Cats are fastidious groomers and if they stop it only takes a day or so for the hair to clump and look oily. And he's dehydrated – dangerously so. But worst of all, I don't like the smell of his breath.'

'They spoil him with fish...'

'No, it's not that. You're right of course, cats often have fishy breath. But this is the smell of urea.' I paused and hung my head with foreboding. 'I'm pretty sure his kidneys have failed.'

I let it sink in, but in truth I was a little puzzled. Boddy was still pleasantly plump, and evidently healthy prior to his sudden-onset illness. Kidney failure is not uncommon in older cats, yet it is neither a weakness, nor, usually, the beginning of the story. There was some information missing, some unknown critical factor at play.

As any cat lover knows, cats are special. They outdo us primates. At a very basic level, mammals only need two-thirds of one kidney, which is why it is possible, if healthy, to donate a whole kidney. To be accurate, a kidney is not really a single organ, but the geometrical result of packing hundreds of thousands of mini-organs, called nephrons, radially and three-dimensionally around a drainage hub, the opening to the ureter, which pipes the urine into the bladder. It is one of nature's many perfect mathematical arrangements.

When uniform damage throughout these nephrons reaches the equivalent of that critical two-thirds loss of functionality, the effects begin to tell. But cats have evolved out of the desert, and there is a touch of the camel about them. Cats' urine is often concentrated to specific gravities that we would consider symbolic of dehydration. They in effect distil the kidney filtrate to reabsorb and reutilise the water, just as we can do, but with far greater evolved ability. You will hardly see a fit, young cat drink at all, except perhaps milk; but then milk is a tasty treat.

The upshot is that a cat's kidneys very rarely simply fail; they compensate. So much so that vets don't call the condition kidney failure, but chronic kidney disease or renal insufficiency, and stage it 1 to 4, 4 being end stage. Usually, a cat would advance through the stages over time, and it would be symptomatically apparent because of increased thirst and loss of body mass.

Boddy was still a large, well-fleshed cat with an overcoat of fat. He looked as if he had skipped all the initial stages and jumped to stage 4. It didn't quite add up.

Matt frowned. Over his shoulder his subordinate bit his lip. This was not the news they wanted to hear. Matt shook his head. 'Dear oh dear,' he said, a little unmilitarily. 'Kidneys.' He considered for a moment. 'Is there anything you can do?'

'It depends. Sometimes, but only sometimes, it's secondary to a primary illness and we can reverse the problem with a drip, but we need to take a blood sample and find out how advanced it is. The kidneys are basically non-regenerative. Once they've gone, they've gone. In human terms it would be a question of dialysis while waiting for a transplant. But in cats...' I trailed off. In cats it happened to be a subject of ethical controversy raging through the august veterinary institutions of the UK. Vets in the USA were popping in transplants without a whiff of moral ambiguity as if planting potatoes – cynically, one would say, for the easy money – but in the UK, my governing body, the Royal College of Veterinary Surgeons, was wrangling with the welfare rights of the donor cat. How could it sign a consent form?

'You see,' Matt continued imploringly as if he hadn't heard me, 'Boddy's a legend. If he dies, the girls in the control tower will be devastated.' He looked away and his eyes were glistening. Not just the girls then. It was comforting to see such compassion in a services officer.

How much of a legend Boddy was I had no idea, but I was about to find out.

Blood sampling – even for vet services – called upon the extremely helpful laboratory technicians of the King Edward VII Memorial Hospital. The next day was Liberation Day, an important public holiday, and I needed the results back so that I had some idea what I was fighting. Time was of the essence. I clipped up Boddy's neck, exposed his jugular vein, and drew off a syringe-full of blood. Next, Sares clamped his leg while I shaved and nicked the skin, pumped up the reluctant vein, and slid in a blue catheter, then I connected a giving set plugged into a warmed bag of Hartmann's solution – a blend of life-sustaining electrolytes – and set the drip rate. He was the perfect patient, cooperative and calm, a real old gentleman of a cat.

The hospital was as industrious and efficient as ever. By evening I was reading a fax with a sinking heart. The figures were not bad; they were terminal. It was indeed full-blown, stage 4 kidney failure at its worst. But I have seen some strange things in my time and even made the occasional unexpected save, so rightly or wrongly I gave Boddy the benefit of the doubt. I was on duty anyway over the midweek holiday and therapy was already underway. I flushed his catheter, set the drip rate by counting 'Mississippis', shut up the surgery for the night and stepped out of the door into a raging blizzard.

THE FEATHERED BICORNE HAT

Liberation Day dawned, and Boddy was no better.

He sat in his cage with a vacant look, barely responding to my strokes and pussy-cat banter. I mixed up some liquid food and syringed it into his mouth, then rearranged his giving set to make him more comfortable. He gave a feeble spluttering purr as I rubbed him under the chin. The litter tray had been used, which was a good sign that I was purging his poison, and the drip was still going in at a slow but steady rate. These things can't be rushed. I planned to resample him the next day when the lab was back at work; the results would determine his fate.

Liberation Day in the Falkland Islands is a day of celebration and remembrance, a drawing together of a community, and a recollection of what might have been; a day, really, for counting one's blessings. And a day when everyone can put down their tools, relax, and raise a glass to freedom. I have never felt so patriotic as I did that day in the Falklands.

This particular Liberation Day marked twenty-four years since the Argentinian invasion of the Falklands – the Conflict – ended, and yet it was still as fresh in the minds of the islanders as if it were yesterday. The reminders were all around, constantly needling. The civilian death toll had been just three, one of them the wife of the serving vet, tragically killed by friendly fire when the Royal Navy bombarded Stanley, but on top of the three were the deaths of 255 British servicemen and some 650 Argentinians. The islanders were and still are undyingly grateful for the sacrifices made by service personnel, without which undoubtedly many more civilians would have perished.

For the invading Argentinians, Stanley's generous harbour, long, ragged coastline, fields of dunes and long white sandy beaches provided simply too many landing points for a relieving force.

Expecting to be besieged by Great Britain's approaching flotilla and with time on their hands to prepare, they mined every possible approach. In my time in the early-2000s, 117 minefields were still active, mainly around Goose Green and the Stanley peninsula, and they have only recently been cleared. Yet despite such obstacles and the traditionally appalling weather,

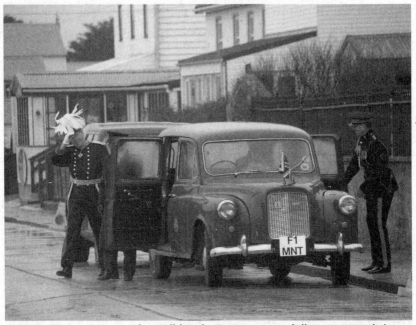

The Falklands Governor, in full ceremonial dress,
arrives for the Liberation Day service

on 14 June 1982, after fierce battles in the hills around Stanley, General Mario Menéndez surrendered to Major General Jeremy Moore of the Royal Marines.

Liberation Day is one week off the southern hemisphere's midwinter, and it was all too readily apparent. An endless barrage of squalls was assaulting Stanley, and successive brutal deposits of sleet had packed and set into a thick and treacherous crackling of ice. But it was appropriate, a fractional illustration of what the British servicemen had had to endure, yomping for miles across the bogs, burdened with kit.

I cleaned Boddy's gummy eyes, rubbed his ears and promised to return later in the afternoon. A Service of Thanksgiving was well underway in Stanley's Christ Church Cathedral. Down by the public jetty I sat in the Rover and listened to the service being broadcast on FIRS, the local radio station. The cathedral was only 200 metres away along the waterfront, and when I wound down the window, I could faintly hear the singing, hauntingly out of phase with the broadcast.

There was a lesson read by the Governor, a dedication of the standard of the Falklands Royal Marines Association, and a moving address about the hardships of the Conflict and the sacrifice of life. Then my heart was stirred by a rendition of my favourite hymn, 'For Those in Peril on the Sea'. Well, actually, 'Eternal Father Strong to Save', but who knows it by that title except clerics and pedants?

Stepping out of the Rover, I walked along Ross Road towards the cathedral, a towering Victorian melange of pale stone and red brick with a heavily buttressed clock tower beneath a pyramidal spire of corrugated iron. The road was windswept and deserted, except for a solitary policeman and a burgundy Hansom cab parked outside the cathedral gate. The cab was spotless, buffed to a glassy shine, with the Royal Coat of Arms on the door panels and a small Union Jack fluttering on the bonnet. The number plate was exclusively brief: FI MNT. The Governor.

A chauffeur in an Oxford-blue uniform and peaked cap hastened from the cathedral, looking slightly hassled. He wrestled with the rear door and held it open against the buffeting wind. A magnificently attired figure with a head of dancing feathers thrust its way through the swaying branches of the cathedral's cypress trees. At that very moment a mussel smacked into the road with a sharp crack and the figure jerked like a puppet. Not an assassin's bullet, but a dolphin gull, now flapping in a quandary overhead trying to decide whether to retrieve it, having used its customary trick to smash open its armour-plated snack. The only onlooker, I stifled a laugh.

The Governor, Howard Pearce, looked every bit the man he was meant to be, in full, bedazzling fig as befitting his lofty station. He was, after all, the direct representative of the Queen, and therefore of HM Government. Only in the Falkland Islands is the governor's uniform seen not as a symbol of colonial repression, but of freedom and patriotism, which is why it is now also the only British Overseas Territory where it is still worn. It is pomp at its most deliciously outrageous.

He was tightly buttoned into a jet-black double-breasted jacket with red cuffs merging into white gloves, the Maltese cross of the CMG prominent on the centre of his chest; two rows of highly polished buttons shone and flashed down his front like landing lights; the gilded hilt of a dress sword swung and glittered in its waxed leather scabbard from a broad, plaited silver belt over red-beribboned trousers; and the silver vermicelli of ornately woven braid glossed his every prominence. But the *pièce de résistance*, the caviar on the sashimi, the hatter's two fingers to the baseball cap, was a quite fantastic flourish of costumery: a black bicorne hat with a fountain of waving swan feathers, worn Nelson-fashion, fore and aft.

He gripped the point of the hat single-handedly as if gently lifting a baby and, removing it from his head, ducked low into the cab. He later confided that one of the feathers was causing him concern.

Each swan feather was actually a pair, skilfully grafted together to create a longer and more impressive 'super-feather' from some fictional giant bird. I suppose peacock feathers would have been a bit proletarian. One of these tantalising creations, the dying art of some octogenarian Savile Row tailor no doubt, had begun to gyrate frantically on its moorings and work itself loose. It had been in imminent danger of plucking itself out and flying off down the harbour to join the steamer ducks. Just as well it didn't. If it had, I'm sure I would have bounded along the foreshore after it like an excitable spaniel chasing a pheasant.

A huddled crowd had gathered at the Liberation Monument below Thatcher Drive and the Secretariat. Paid for by public subscription, the monument bears testimony to those who lost their lives in the Conflict. Generally, this sort of creation has a tendency towards dry grimness, a reflection of the reality of war perhaps, but the 1982 Liberation Monument is a fine work of craftsmanship, an imaginative and uplifting addition to the historic heart of the waterfront.

The dead are listed on bronze panels depicting scenes from the war, and a stout granite obelisk is topped by a magnificent Britannia. She stands tall in a tunic of armoured scales over flowing robes, helmeted head gazing defiantly heavenward, a shield carelessly propped against her thigh, her arm stretched high on the shaft of a purposeful trident. And the face: piercing gaze, hawkish nose, headmistress eyes. More than a hint of the Iron Lady. No coincidence then that the road is named Thatcher Drive.

A parade of soldiers bearing arms and standards, support- ed by a brass band, marched gamely through the biting wind and scurries of snow, and lined up in front of the monument. Reverend Sweeting, surplice flailing in the gusts, conducted a Service of Remembrance. The Governor, the Commander of the British Forces of the South Atlantic Islands, representatives from each of the three services, and a variety of other interested parties laid wreaths of poppies, their shoulders dusted with snowflakes. A bugler, frozen lips on frozen mouthpiece, somehow played the 'Last Post', the long mournful notes saddening the soul as the comfortless pewter waves frothed and foamed behind him. During the minute of silence that followed, I looked about at the bowed heads and pale faces and felt unexpectedly moved. In the UK, the Falklands War is a footnote in history, the last quaint twitch of a fallen empire. In the islands, it is still fresh and alive, a deep font of patriotism. There had been fear, there had been death, and there had been triumph. There was still the threat, albeit diluted.

The 'Reveille' broke the spell and roused the crowd. The sombre mood was swept aside by a buzz of eager anticipation for the civic reception in the barn-like hall of the Falkland Island Defence Force, with unlimited free drink laid on by the government. After the morning's solemn acts of remembrance, the remainder of Liberation Day is a strongly alcoholic affair.

Not for me, though: I was on duty. I went up to the hall and joined the packed crowd, shook hands with the Governor, then struggled out into the worsening weather, ice pricking my eyes. An ancient, shrunken woman with tousled grey hair and red-veined cheeks lurched towards me in a thin dress, blissfully unaware of the stinging cold. She swung a plastic beer cup in the vague direction of my face.

'I have just one thing...' – she raised a wavering finger to emphasise her proclamation – '...just one thing to say...' The plastic cup was thrust up my nose. 'Here's to freedom.'

Yes, I thought. Yes indeed. 'Here's to freedom!' I replied, only not too well; my throat seemed strangely choked.

EYES TO THE SKIES

Back at the clinic Boddy was showing no improvement at all. Quite the opposite. An intravenous drip is a sort of poor man's dialysis, relying heavily on some residual kidney function to do all the necessary filtering and sorting. The litter tray was swimming in urine, yet Boddy was still dehydrated. This could only mean one thing: no ability to concentrate. His kidneys were now gushing taps.

I have never lost my awe of evolutionary engineering – we are still second-rate copiers of nature's designs – and the kidney is a masterpiece. At the head of each nephron is the glomerulus, a tiny acorn cup that embraces a ball of capillaries and sieves out an initial filtrate like coffee from the grounds. This fluid is the basis of urine, but not before its passage along the convoluted tubule to the core of the kidney, during which alchemy occurs. The fluid is processed, and far from being mechanical and passive, this processing is proactive, juggling and exchanging minerals and electrolytes, sorting and discarding toxins, and regulating water loss. The kidneys are capable of distilling the urine to a concentration far in excess of the blood stream. They even regulate blood pressure, command the heart and govern red blood cell production. And all this in response to a set of finely tuned, inter-regulating chemical messengers and activators.

But its superlative design also highlights the kidney's one weakness: a virtual inability to regenerate. Imagine a building of intense and delicate design, with architecture so compact, so intertwining, that it could only exist by raising it up from the foundation stone. Rather like Gaudi's peerless Sagrada Familia in Barcelona. Attempting to treat a failed kidney is like blowing that building apart and trying to patch it up with concrete: it becomes a mere simulacrum.

Boddy had reached that point. His pitiful expression and toxic breath said it all. Nonetheless, I took a blood sample. I always feel the need to know just how badly a case has gone awry and add it to the stock of experience. Boddy's fate chattered out of the fax machine within the hour.

I was incredulous. Before the treatment, his figures were about as bad as I had ever seen. They had now virtually doubled.

I could not recall such spectacular kidney failure, besides which an intravenous drip nearly always at least dilutes the toxins, even if temporarily. Something still didn't add up. But sadly for Boddy, mystery or not, there was only one humane course of action. I made the dreaded phone call, and then, very gently for a very gentle cat, put him to sleep. Finally, in the endless pursuit of a diagnosis, I removed a tiny fragment of his kidney with a Tru-Cut biopsy needle.

Air traffic control had one request: that before rigor mortis set in, we curled him up as if napping on a chair, his repose for the celestial air traffic control tower – guiding in pussy cat angels, no doubt.

The next day Matt collected his body. 'We're going to miss him,' he said. 'Boddy was always around and yet he never got in the way. Everyone's friend.' He put his shoulder to the door and

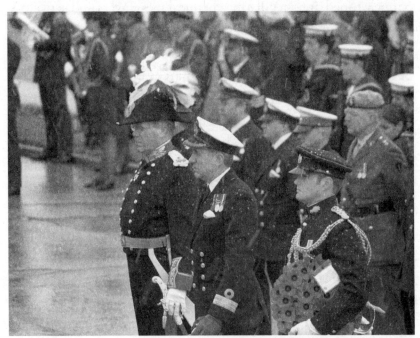

Falklands Liberation Day ceremonies

pushed out into the wind. 'The funeral's at lunchtime by the way. Eyes to the skies.'

'Eyes to the... what...?'

'The boys are giving him a flypast. I've cleared it with the CO.'

Perhaps I was still a bit emotional from Liberation Day, or perhaps I am just a soft touch for gestures of affection towards animal companions, but I felt deeply moved. The Mount Pleasant Complex was there to deploy, if called upon, its full ferocious might. It was manned by professional servicemen trained to kill. But so long as the hint of humanity still existed – such as kindness towards animals – civilisation prevailed.

Sure enough at lunchtime there was a rumble in the skies like distant rolling thunder. Sares and I ran outside.

'Do you know what we call that?' Sares asked, hugging her shoulders against the cold.

'Noise pollution?'

She fixed me with a look of infinite patience. I was a hopeless case. 'No! We actually call it the Sound of Freedom.'

'Really? Oh – I rather like that.'

Through the clouds above Stanley we could glimpse three Tornados shadowed by a VC-10. 'And they,' said Sares, pointing skywards, 'are Faith, Hope and Charity.'

RAF 1435 Flight, the Falklands' airborne defence unit, has an illustrious history. It was formed during the Second World War to assist in the defence of Malta using Spitfires, a tough posting with a low probability of survival. By tradition their jets still sport the Maltese cross and bear the names of the three original Gloster Gladiators the Spitfires replaced: Faith, Hope and Charity. Later, deployed to the Falklands, a fourth reserve jet was added to the flight, and with typical RAF tongue-in-cheek humour it was named... Desperation.

This flypast was not some flagrant waste of taxpayers' money. Just as Olympic athletes can ill afford to slacken in their training, so too must jet fighter pilots hurl themselves about the skies on an almost daily basis to keep their skills razor sharp. The flypast was simply a good way of making a practice run purposeful, of saluting a fine regimental mascot and boosting morale. Who would begrudge Boddy that?

Oddly though, very oddly – and how could I possibly know? – as I gazed up at the planes, I was looking at the solution to his perplexing case.

COOL FOR CATS

In the evening, I was driving out on the MPA road to join a team of my colleagues at the government farm, Saladero, where an ovine embryo transfer programme was in full swing. I had struck up a friendship with Dr Frans Jooste, the reproduction consultant, and he was going to teach me how to flush and collect embryos from super-ovulated ewes. It was a rare opportunity to gain some specialist knowledge, a masterclass in juggling baby lambs.

The road, mostly gravel and dangerous at the best of times, was thickly capped with polished ice, but at least the skies had finally cleared. The Land Rover had a tendency to yaw and sway at unexpected intervals, so I was pootling along at a genteel pace, absorbing the sounds of Forces Radio. The broadcaster, Hermina Graham, suddenly mentioned Boddy's name. Intrigued, I pulled over onto the cambered edge and listened as I stared up at Wickham Heights, resplendent in snow lit burnt orange by the sinking sun.

She was sad, she said, to report the death of a legendary cat: Sergeant Boddington – a patient and stalwart companion of all those who passed through air traffic control and the

Met Office. The funeral had been held directly in front of the Control Tower, where he was laid to rest in a small coffin during a short service. Eyes filled and cheeks were wiped as the boys of 1435 Flight did him proud with a low flypast in tight formation. One Tornado peeled away and disappeared into the ether, a manoeuvre called 'the missing man' which honours the loss of one of their number. Words were said, and the hole was filled and marked with a cross. He would be sorely missed by all.

'And so', she finished, 'the next hour is dedicated to the cat that gave unstintingly of his companionship. This track is for Sergeant Boddington, late of air traffic control, who was put to sleep today at the ripe old age of sixteen. May he rest in peace.'

It was 'Cool for Cats' by Squeeze.

Perfect.

I'm unashamed to admit my eyes brimmed with emotion.

TORNADOS ON ICE

A week later an officer from the Mount Pleasant Met Office came into the surgery with a cat for a routine vaccination. 'So, who's this?' I enquired, eyeing the box with curiosity.

The officer unclipped the lid and pulled out a floppy ginger cat. I could scarcely believe my eyes. 'My god, but it's Boddy!'

He placed the cat on the table. 'Almost,' he replied enigmatically. 'Actually, it's Crusty, Boddy's littermate. We think he's a real twin.'

I could feel myself grinning from ear to ear. 'I had no idea he even existed. Does he have Boddy's same good disposition?'

'Identical in every respect... but even lazier.'

I gave him a routine health check prior to the vaccination. 'Very healthy. In excellent order for a cat of sixteen, much the same as I imagine Boddy was before he was struck down by his illness.'

'Yes,' he said. 'That was all very sad. Any idea what happened to him?'

I shrugged in defeat. 'Apart from kidney failure? No, not really. There's a reason for everything, but I guess we'll never know.'

So that was that – had it not been for one chance comment.

Air traffic control was far too quiet and lonely without Boddy, and they made it known that they would be happy to take on an appropriate cat. Such a cat came along in need of a loving and caring home, a friendly young tabby-and-white female called Diddle. Four servicewomen came in from MPA to collect her, among them Flight Lieutenant Ali Caper, whom I had met when I was stuck in Fox Bay.

'It's been terrible without Boddy,' she said. 'He was such a presence. The tower's been deathly.' She reminisced about the flypast and described the neatly marked grave, and how Boddy, before he fell ill, had developed a new habit of visiting the mess down the runway for a few extra treats.

My ears pricked up. The unsolved case still bothered me and here was a line of reasoning I had completely neglected. I was thinking: runway... contaminants... the impeccable habits of cats...

'He was a strange case, Ali. I've never known kidneys to be so suddenly and devastatingly destroyed. He clearly had no problems before, he was in superb condition: plump, well fed, glossy. Something happened, something to do with MPA. I guess the runway is covered in aviation fuel?'

'No, no,' said Ali, aghast at the very idea of such carelessness. 'Not avgas. Well, maybe a little. But under the present conditions they've been spraying heavily with ICA.' She giggled. 'The trouble with the Tornados is they kind of figure skate.'

'ICA?'

'Yes, ice control agent. Antifreeze. The conditions have been appallingly icy, and they've been using it by the tankerload. Can't have millions of pounds' worth of valuable hardware shooting off the end of the runway.'

'Antifreeze!' I blurted out. 'Bloody antifreeze!'

She took a step back as if for safety.

'Ali, it's the antifreeze. Ethylene glycol. It destroys kidneys. Cats wouldn't choose to lick it, but they'll always groom themselves, paws and all. ICA killed Boddy.'

The light dawned. 'Ah.' Ali's face shone with understanding. 'And although he lived there for years,' she went on slowly, 'his traipsing down to the mess was a recent habit – and they've been using more antifreeze than normal. I know the Dog Section is banned from the runway...' She struck her forehead with her palm. 'That's why they ban the dogs!'

'Yes. Dogs especially. They like the taste.'

Ethylene glycol obliterates the kidneys by crystallising in the tubules. Meticulous Boddy, after calling in at the mess for a tidbit or two, had padded along the runway and returned to the control tower only to find something sticky and sweet coating his paws, whereupon, like any self-respecting cat, he had licked them back to perfection – poisoning himself in the process.

I still had the sample, so I sent it off. When the pathology results came back they were unequivocal. A photomicrograph showed dark renal tubules crammed with incongruous, brightly reflective crystals: calcium oxalate. The report read: 'Morphologic diagnosis: acute ethylene glycol toxicity'.

Boddy's fate was all down to figure-skating Tornados.

There was little that could have been done, but at least Boddy's loss was Diddle and Crusty's gain. Lesson learned, the control tower crew instigated 'cat-meandering suppression measures' during freezing weather when the runway was being de-iced, thus ensuring that all cherished felines' kidneys remained fully sound and functional.

It was Boddy's gift.

That, I reasoned, was a worthy sacrifice.

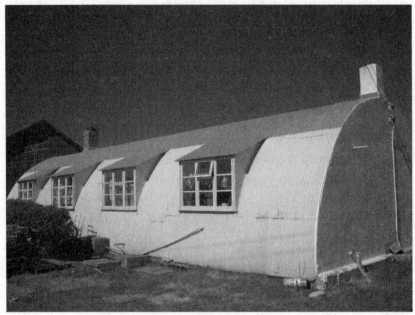

One of the many different architectural styles of Stanley, this one a home converted from a Nissan hut

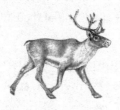

THE LAST REINDEER

Sir Edward.B.Binnie Esq, South Georgia Nov:11th 1911

Act Stipendiary Magistrate,

<u>South Georgia.</u>

Sir,

I have the honour to inform you that my brother, who is Manager of the Ocean Whaling Co:,and I have imported here to South Georgia 10 Reindeer (3 bulls and 7 cows) as these thrive very well in the cold region of the North, I feel sure that they will thrive and become prolific in time,if they are left alone,which would most assuredly be an asset to South Georgia.

I would deem it a great obligement if an order could be issued for their protection.

Awaiting the favour of your reply

I have the honour to remain,Sir,

yours respectfully,

C.A.LARSEN

Letter from Carl Larsen to Sir Edward Binnie:
British Antarctic Survey Archives, ref LS7/3/7

GUNS AND HARPOONS

It began with a nuclear disaster.

No... let's go back further. Whalers. It began with whalers. More specifically, Norwegian whalers, performing gruelling work in gruelling conditions and hankering for something comforting from home. Namely, a spot of hunting, but with rifles rather than harpoons, and with the reward of a fresh, juicy venison steak instead of the staple greasy seal or whale meat, sluiced down, no doubt, with generous slugs of fiery aquavit.

Thankfully, whaling is now all but consigned to history – at least on the grand scale – yet the undeniable truth of the matter is that the rendered blubber of not just whales, but seals and penguins too, literally oiled the cogs and lit the lamps of the Industrial Revolution. The modern oil industry was then embryonic, confined to curiosities such as tar pits and strange, flammable seepages in desert sands. Without whaling and all its repugnant commerce, we would not be who we are today. We owe whales a great deal.

Scandinavian sailors, thanks to their long tradition of harvesting whale products locally, were at the heart of industrialised international whaling as it emerged in the nineteenth century. The Norwegians were hardy to the core and used to the bone-breaking toil, rank odours and brutal vicissitudes of the fishing industry. Among them was Carl Larsen. He must have been an intriguing character, the sort of adventurer with whom I would like to have chewed the fat over a steaming crock of stew – venison perhaps – in the crackling warmth of a log fire, with snow drifting high against the door. He, this one man, was almost certainly key to my involvement with a herd of reindeer more than a century later. This man, and a false economy on a critical piece of nuclear hardware that ended up costing the earth – or at least a good chunk of it.

The pattern of causation that steers our lives is so often buried in time.

Carl Anton Larsen was joint leader on the highly productive Swedish Antarctic Expedition of 1901–03, an expedition not without suffering but which scored several resounding firsts in the annals of Antarctic exploration. They surveyed large tracts of territory, and it was Larsen who found the first fossils on the great white continent, and first skied on the vast ice shelf that now bears his name. But the expedition was driven by a powerful commercial motive: it was also a reconnaissance mission for the whaling industry.

During the expedition they put into a superb harbour on South Georgia, a one-hundred-mile by twenty-mile sticklebacked island in the scribbled shape of a diving fox. South Georgia had been claimed for Great Britain in 1775 by Captain James Cook. Some will know of it as the site of Ernest Shackleton's grave, others perhaps for the landing of Argentinian elite troops thinly and farcically disguised as scrap-metal merchants, the trigger for the Falklands War. It is, by all accounts, quite stunning.

Littering the shore of this natural harbour were the tools of the trade left by a century or more of sealers, notably the bulbous, two-handled cast-iron trypots for 'trying out', that is rendering, blubber. Two of these now sit in my garden in St Helena, more genteelly repurposed as planters for, fittingly, blood-orange cannas. Such death these pots have seen.

The harbour had a safe anchorage with a sheltered pocket of flat land ideal for settlement, and abundant fresh water gushing from the glaciers of the mountainous spine. The Norwegians named it Grytviken, the Bay of Pots, after the trypots. Larsen saw that the southern seas contained untapped riches and knew immediately that this was his natural base. So, in 1904, wasting no time whatsoever, he raised capital, founded the Compañía Argentina de Pesca, the Argentine Fishing Company, obtained a licence from the British authorities, and with extraordinary speed and efficiency along with a hundred or so of his hardies raised the first land-based whaling station on South Georgia at Grytviken.

It was a resounding success, and soon South Georgia became the heart of the whaling industry, with further stations such as Prince Olav Harbour, Godthul and Husvik proclaiming their obvious Scandinavian provenance.

The aesthetically pleasing coat of arms of South Georgia and the South Sandwich Islands bears a shield with the classic imperial lion rampant, supported on one side by a fur seal on a plinth of rock and on the other by a macaroni penguin on a slice of ice. All quite appropriate. Above, forming the crest on a visored helmet, a hoof perched on each of four small mountain pinnacles, stands a regal and superbly antlered reindeer bull. Totally inappropriate, any zoologist not in the know might comment.

Reindeer, or caribou, are to the Arctic what penguins are to the Antarctic: icons of their respective global extremities. Never the twain shall meet. Surely everyone knows that? To have a penguin and a reindeer on the same territorial coat of arms seems laughable.

But Larsen realised that what works in the north *could* work in the south. He gazed at the vegetated pediments of the steep glaciated ridges, the lichen-embossed rocks and the coastal flats fertilised by seal and penguin guano and thick with nutritious tussac grass, and he saw the opportunity to provide his men with a pressure valve: reindeer hunting. So, in 1911, he brought down three males and seven females from Norway and established what became known as the Barff herd, planting the seed for one of the most challenging experiences of my veterinary career. And the most rewarding.

A further introduction in 1912 ended in disaster when the whole herd was buried in an avalanche. But in 1925 a third introduction established the Busen herd, separated from their cousins by the ice barriers of glaciers reaching down into the sea.

Sixty years later, a catastrophe on the other side of the globe was to give the herds a status beyond mere geographical curiosity.

MELTDOWN

In 1986 I was working at my first practice, Bainbridge & Butt, in Wellingborough, an old shoe-factory town on the north bank of the River Nene in Northamptonshire. Because of the former tanneries discharging their effluent onto the flood plains, it also happens to be notorious as the 'anthrax incubator belt of Britain', which was how, incidentally – and a little strangely – I got the job; almost certainly the only favour anthrax ever did anyone.

Run by highly experienced partners, it was an excellent mixed practice for grounding my university-acquired knowledge, having a healing hoof in almost every veterinary field: horses, pigs, cattle, sheep, and goats, along with all the pets of a sprawling Midlands town.

But we also did export abattoir work.

This was my least favourite task. To supervise the slaughter of a thousand lambs a day and slap my authority four times on each carcass with my purple EEC stamp – buttock, buttock, shoulder, shoulder, endlessly, endlessly in the dripping, dank, cavernous chillers – was not what I aspired to, not what I had trained for; but it was contracted out by the local council and provided a rich stream of income for the practice.

On the wall of the meat inspectors' office was a map of the United Kingdom, large parts of which were marked in red: Wales, Scotland, the Pennines, the Lake District and so on, all areas of high rainfall. These red zones were 'no take' for sheep, for the very good reason that they had been irradiated by nuclear fallout, and meat that pings on a Geiger counter is not recommended as part of a healthy diet.

A few weeks earlier, on the night of 26 April 1986, several miles from the city of Pripyat in Soviet Ukraine, a poorly prepared night shift undertook a safety test on one of Russia's RBMK-1000 nuclear reactors at the Vladimir Ilyich Lenin Nuclear Power Plant. The test scenario sought to answer a question which in hindsight is steeped in irony: what would happen in the event of a power outage? As safety tests go, it could not have been less safe. Chernobyl was the world's worst nuclear disaster, emitting a plume of isotopes into the atmosphere with something of the order of 400 times the radioactivity of Hiroshima. The fallout settled over circumpolar regions and a large swathe of Western Europe. I remember staring at the red hatchings on the office wall map with stupefaction; it underlined the absolute futility of nuclear conflict (still on the table in the dying days of the Cold War) - no wonder it's referred to as MAD, Mutually Assured Destruction. More to the point for this story, as the rain fell and the dust settled, all the reindeer of the northern hemisphere in their high snowy latitudes, and therefore theoretically in the world, were irradiated.

Only, thanks to Larsen, that wasn't quite the case.

The Norwegian reindeer of South Georgia, safe from nuclear fallout at the opposite end of the globe, were spared. They were also, since Carl Larsen had left them to their own devices, breeding well. Rather too well, in fact. They had bred into their thousands. Wherein lay another problem.

South Georgia is a nature sanctuary, home to colonies of birds and mammals whose numbers are staggering: some 7 million penguins, 2 million fur seals, half a million elephant seals, and well over 10 million other seabirds. The two herds of reindeer occupied one third of South Georgia's vegetated area and they were overgrazing the land, so severely in fact that the herds were suffering a 30–40 per cent annual mortality rate, largely due to starvation and to the desperate animals falling off cliffs while reaching for food. Their splayed, four-toed hooves are designed to help them snowshoe across the flat Arctic tundra; they are not mountain goats.

In addition, their natural migrations ranging as far as 700 miles to seek out food were impossible to imitate in South Georgia's terrain, riven as it is by murderous gorges blocked by barriers of sea and ice. The animals were trapped and suffering. They were also transforming the landscape, destroying the habitat of the local wildlife: as the protective maze of tall pedestals of tussac grass was overgrazed, the fertile soil between, manured by hordes of breeding creatures over millennia, was being washed out to sea. It was a welfare and ecological timebomb set ticking by human meddling. There was only one remedy: to turn back the clock.

It was decided to eradicate the reindeer.

TOO MANY SKELETONS

Vic Epstein stormed into my box room of an office, his brow beetling in consternation: 'Joe, we have a problem!' I had learned to trust and admire him even if I still found him hard to like. Behind his abrasive Australian manner lay a shrewd, analytical mind that cut cleanly through the murk of indecision.

'We do?'

'Yup. Our reindeer are dying.'

I asked the obvious question. 'What reindeer, Vic? Do we have reindeer?' It was firmly set in my mind that a reindeer's place was alongside the Inuit and polar bears in the icy north, yet here we were most definitely off the tip of South America.

'Sure we have,' he replied as if it was blatantly obvious. 'They brought them up from South Georgia at a cost of almost a quarter of a mill and now they're dying. The farmer just phoned to say there's only fourteen left.' He shook his head in sad disbelief and lowered his tone. 'Four months ago, he had over thirty. We need to account for them and find out what the hell's happening before we lose them all. Each animal's now worth over £15,000. We're gonna have to make a plan and get over there.'

I tackled Sares; she was my go-to spiritual and practical guide for everything Falklands. She filled me in over lunch.

'It was a big deal, Joe, and cost the government something like £200,000. Tim Bonner and a team went all the way to Alaska to get training in herding and handling reindeer. Then they hired a fisheries patrol vessel, loaded it with capture pens and feed, went down to South Georgia and caught a bunch of reindeer calves.'

'Calves?'

'Yes. Easier to handle, easier to domesticate, and take up less space. They reckon the adults would have gone bonkers. It could have been a welfare situation. Anyways... they brought them up here and put them on the government farm at Saladero. But they didn't get it all quite right and some of them died, so they fenced off Rapid Point and shifted them there.'

We pored over a contour map. Rapid Point lay on the north coast of West Falkland in an area called West Lagoons not far from the farming settlement of Hill Cove. It was an undulating, roughly oval peninsula of land attached to the mainland by a narrow swampy neck, ideally suited for isolating with a nine-foot-high deer fence to create an area of some 1,500 acres.

'Two hundred thousand, Sares.' I whistled. 'That's a truck-load of money. But why? Why bother?'

'Because of Chernobyl. They reckon they're the only reindeer in the world that didn't have their genes cooked. And because there's a plan to eradicate them from South Georgia. They're doing too much damage there. And then again, because one day in the future, instead of going out for a boring old beef steak, we can stuff our bellies with fresh local venison.' She smiled, all cheery freckles and blazing hair.

It was this and more. The South Georgia reindeer were direct descendants of the true wild European reindeer and had been sourced from one of their last refuges, the central mountains of Norway in the region of Hemsedal. It was the opinion of the scientific community that conserving the last and only un-Chernobylised – a term that could only belong to our crazy nuclear age – reindeer genome was not just desirable, but a moral obligation.

On top of that, the Falkland Islands Government could, like Larsen, see some potential in farming them. The Falkland Islands had already been irrevocably altered by the presence of man and beast, and land was both plentiful and varied, the wildlife areas protected. This was not the pristine wilderness of South Georgia, so why not introduce reindeer? Organic reindeer steaks would sell for a healthy premium to visiting tourists and the stream of cruise ships en route to the Antarctic Peninsula, and there was a possible side industry in antler bone for souvenirs and knife handles, let alone valuable antler velvet for its dubious and unsubstantiated medicinal properties – a booming and lucrative market that, no matter how intense one's scepticism, it would be rash to ignore.

'The fly in the ointment,' Sares continued, raising a well-tended eyebrow, 'is Jérôme Poncet.'

The Frenchman Jérôme Poncet was a shrewd and clever scientist, and a brilliantly skilled Antarctic yachtsman. After the government initiative to translocate reindeer, he had grasped the same opportunity by twice sailing down to South Georgia to bring back calves in a pen on the deck of his yacht, *Golden Fleece*, which he then allowed to roam free on his private island off West Falkland, and all for a fraction of the cost. Everyone lauded his success, but it was also rather humiliating for the government. And he knew it.

It was abundantly clear that there, on Beaver Island, the reindeer were booming. Jérôme was not a huge fan of the British authorities but, whether by dint of good husbandry or lucky bravado, he had pulled it off where we had not, and there were lessons that could be usefully learned, rather than wastefully discarded in a fit of pique. Why did his reindeer prosper while ours died? It had to be to do with habitat.

'Oh, and there's something else you should know. They tried to catch the reindeer last year. They went out to Rapid Point with motorbikes and even had the *Tamar* standing offshore to take them away, but the reindeer ran them ragged, and then...' she pursed her lips with supressed amusement, 'they jumped into the sea. Apparently, reindeer can swim – rather well.'

I mentally logged my first lesson: use a softly, softly approach. They must be courted, loved and lulled.

'What was the plan though, Sares? Where was the ship going to take them?'

'Ah, just the best place. Albemarle – Cape Meredith – the southernmost point of West Falkland. It's wild, Joe. Wild, stark and beautiful. And one of the best farmers, Leon Berntsen. We were going to split the herd to double our chances of success, and a couple of years ago, he deer-fenced a whole area called the Three Crowns. He's desperate to get the reindeer. Oh, and Joe...' She paused again, knowing I was easily drawn. 'He has a lighthouse. Well, more of a beacon really. But it's old and I think you'd like it.'

Sares knew, thanks to my frequent visits to the rusting, windswept lighthouse at Cape Pembroke, decommissioned in 1982 and battered by the prevailing westerlies, that from childhood I had had a slight obsession with lighthouses and beacons. The dazzling sweep of the Eddystone Lighthouse perched on a reef seventeen miles out to sea could be seen from the clifftop of my village. Lighthouses are to me one of the greatest of all architectural feats, absurd skinny towers on godforsaken pinnacles of ocean-blasted rock, designed to resist the irrepressible forces of nature at their angriest and most extreme. Stubbornly, against all the odds, they succeed and have saved and continue to save thousands of lives as a result. Red, white, steel or granite, raised on trestles or piled on a rock, I love their diversity and I love their ingenuity.

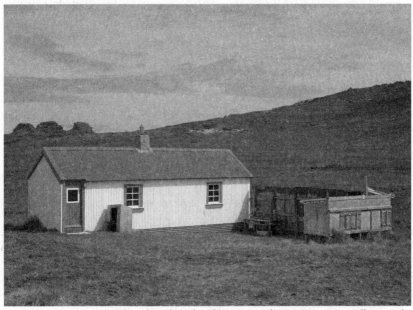

The shepherd's shanty at Three Crowns, Albemarle

Reindeer and a beacon. And as it turned out, no ordinary beacon. What an outrageously unique combination. If I wanted to save the reindeer and have the opportunity to explore an outlandishly placed beacon, there was only one way forward: do my research and know the beast.

Rangifer tarandus aka reindeer aka caribou, from the native American language Mi'kmaq, meaning 'snow shoveller'. Reindeer lichen, *Cladonia rangiferina*, their absolute ambrosia. Second to that, mosses. Also partial to grasses, leaves, mushrooms, bird eggs, seaweed and an occasional side dish of lemming – which must come as a shock to the unsuspecting lemming, happy and secure in the company of ostensible herbivores. Range circumpolar in the extreme north of the Americas and Eurasia. Fourteen subspecies, the Norwegian mountain reindeer being one of the genetically purest. Norwegian... ah, now the project started to make sense.

Specialised cloven hooves, four toes, two large and two small, hard in winter for gripping the ice, soft and spongy in summer for the thawing tundra and mossy taiga. Unlike all other deer, antlers on both genders. Domesticated by the Arctic peoples and critical for their existence as beasts of burden, sledge pullers and a source of food and clothing. Predated on by the brown bear, lynx and their ultimate enemy, the wolf, hence a highly developed flight reflex – as I was to experience. All in all, an interesting species.

Then there was the final fact worth noting. Sares was right. Powerful swimmers. The waters off Rapid Point were littered with tiny and not so tiny islets. Maybe they weren't dead. Maybe they had simply migrated.

Vic liked the idea. 'Sares,' he shouted. 'Get us a plane. We're goin' a-deerhuntin'.'

'No problem – I think I can find you a half-decent pilot.' She winked. Troyd, her husband, was the very man.

Troyd gunned the Islander aircraft down the Stanley airstrip, and revved hard to clear the lantern room of the Cape Pembroke lighthouse, which looked like an abandoned chess piece in the sharp sunlight. Then he arced the plane round to head west across the heart of East Falkland.

Stanley lies on the far, fingery tip of East Falkland. As the capital of an archipelago scattered over a challenging expanse of temperamental ocean, its peripheral location seems at first poorly conceived. But in fact, Stanley is there for the very good reason that the site was recommended to the Admiralty by Captain FitzRoy of the *Beagle* when perambulating around the coast with Charles Darwin.

He noted that Port Stanley was the ideal anchorage for the establishment of a settlement because of a confluence of local factors: the alignment of the long, linear double harbours with an eastern approach dominated by the reassuring pushback of the prevailing westerlies (a vessel reliant on sail is otherwise easily driven onto a lee shore); good shelter; and plentiful supplies of peat to fuel the home fires. On still days Stanley Harbour, a long groove in the surrounding landscape, was reputed to cradle the brown smoke of burning peat like a tureen of oxtail soup.

We flew inland, low over the shattered ridges, sage-green hills and boulder-strewn valleys of East Falkland, hopped across the dark dividing waters of the Falkland Sound, and headed to the northern coast of sparsely populated West Falkland.

The two main islands are neatly divided by the diagonal gash of the Sound, their coastlines crowded with thousands of fragments in all shapes, sizes and topographies. Some thrust skyward like Steeple Jason, some are rambling and substantial like Saunders, some low and sandy like Pebble, or cliff-girt like Beauchêne; others are richly varied like Sea Lion. They descend all the way down the scale through uninhabited humble islets the size of playing fields to splinters of wave-lashed rocks. The land has been messily toffee-hammered, but to spectacular effect, and there is no better place to view it than from the sky.

Rapid Point, in contrast, looked sad and drab, a grey-brown club of coast surrounded by a starburst of bald and rounded islets. Troyd tilted the tiny, agile plane and buzzed them all, Vic and I leaning to peer out of the windows. We zig-zagged over Christmas Island and Shallow Bay, then expanded our search to local headlands and out to Keppel Island. There were no hiding places, no escape.

Disappointment pervaded the cabin. 'No bloody reindeer here,' said Vic. 'Let's go look at the real thing. Troyd, can you wing us over the mainland?'

This was my first sight of the herd, indeed my first ever real-life sight of reindeer. They were huddled by the deer fence, a sorry sight, shadows too angular on the tawny ground, flanks hollow and ribs grooved. We counted thirteen – just thirteen survivors out of the fifty-nine our team had shipped back from South Georgia. Vic groaned. 'One less again. They're in trouble all right. Troyd, can we search the Point now?'

The plane swept back and forth over the land, and left us in no doubt what the small white deposits, like the scattered ashes of old campfires, actually represented. Some were ringed by what looked like wind-blown tufts of cotton wool caught in the scrub. Hair.

Vic sighed. 'Well, that's that. Skeletonised remains. We've lost them.'

But that wasn't that. Vic soon despatched me back to Rapid Point armed with a GPS and the government Land Rover we kept at Port Howard. The task: to account for as many reindeer as possible, and to find and map their remains. This was a financial loss for the government, and we were accountable. No matter how uncomfortable, we needed to provide the data.

It was high summer and Rapid Point had only just become accessible across the infamous peat bogs, our small climatic window for action. Even so, I spent one whole joyless afternoon knee deep in peat with un-summery hailstones bouncing off my shoulders as I used every means to extricate the mired Rover. Getting bogged is a national pastime and a rite of passage, but the islanders are escapologists. As an incomer, getting out unaided was the only way to avoid unbridled hilarity and buying everyone a round of drinks. The trick; by the way, is a monkey jack on top of a spare wheel buried in the peat.

The hunt for skeletons was dismal. Every heap of bones saddened me more, not least because I had now met the surviving herd of reindeer with their doleful expressions and hat-rack ribcages and was falling in love with them. Some were clearly heavily pregnant, but with their nutritional state at such a low ebb, any calves born would surely be doomed. Several looked parasitised, with debilitating scours plastering their backsides. Their lives dangled by the finest of threads.

Slowly, to and fro through heather-like diddle-dee and the bizarre green domes of balsam bog, I laid down a thorough search pattern. Some reindeer had crawled away to die and were concealed by overhanging ledges, others had perished on the crown of the land, fully exposed to the elements. Most wretchedly, I found mothers with their calves, their bones pitifully interlocked, the maternal instinct so powerful they had continued to huddle around the corpses of their already deceased young. It's not only humans who mourn.

On the east side of the peninsula, a thin spit of sand and shingle clings to a small triangular remnant called Dutchman's Point. The tide was rising and the waters were about to meet, but my conscience forced me to park up the vehicle and run across anyway.

It was as well. Two more skeletons. I pulled out the GPS, logged the coordinates, then hastily rolled up my jeans to wade back, very nearly cut off by the rising waters. Another round of drinks narrowly avoided.

On a small crescent beach, I found a gruesome monument to masculine aggression: two big-boned skeletons of mature stags locked together in eternal combat, their impressive, many-tined antlers irrevocably entangled. I imagined the prolonged death, head-to-head and eye-to-eye for days on end until thirst and hunger took their toll. As a battle for genetic dominance, it was a Darwinian failure.

I returned to Stanley with a heavy heart, surprised by how profoundly the visit had affected me. It was a pitiful harvest. Furthermore, there was little hope for the survivors, bone rattlers every one of them. I produced a report with the most sorrowful map of my career. It was entitled: 'West Lagoons, Rapid Point, Reindeer Carcass Sites'. I have the map still. It is deceptively pretty. A snow-white peninsula with coffee contours set in a nursery-blue sea with small, black, dendritic strands symbolising giant sea kelp along the shoreline, the whole overlaid by a violet grid. Almost worth framing, were it not for the twenty-four reindeer carcasses, each discretely enumerated, their bleached bones, fear and pain reduced to small, crisp, blood-red dots. A map of the fallen.

There was no escaping the maths. None had swum away, none had drowned and been carried off by ocean currents. They had simply laid down and died.

Vic called me into his office. He had read my report and chewed over its implications. 'Righto,' he said purposefully. 'The reindeer are our number one priority. They're valuable animals and their welfare's at stake. So's ours,' he added drily. He fell silent for a moment, then continued in a quieter, graver voice, running his fingers through his fluffy grey hair as if combing out his thoughts. 'It seems to me we have no option. We must try to move them.'

'It would be for the best,' I replied uncertainly, wriggling to get comfortable in the visitor's chair, a low, armless contraption with misbehaving wheels. 'But if they've started calving, we won't get near them, and if they haven't, the cows may well slip their fawns with the stress of transporting them. It's a long way to Cape Meredith. Damned if we do, damned if we don't.'

'The trouble with you, Joe, is you worry too much. The risk of abortion is unavoidable, but it's that or... well, there's no choice. Either they all die, some die or, if we're bloody lucky, none die. The bogs have dried out and we only have this small window of opportunity. I want you to go back there and see what you can do. Above all, I want you to supervise their welfare every step of the way. We wouldn't normally sanction the transportation of heavily pregnant animals, but when the devil's at the wheel...' He leaned back, kicked out his legs, and smiled supportively. 'Look – just do what you can. I don't expect miracles.'

I found Sares grappling with the drawer of a stubborn filing cabinet. 'Food, Sares, food. What can I tempt reindeer with? Somehow I have to befriend them.' For all her love of *haute couture*, she was a farmgirl at heart.

'OK. What do they eat?'

I told her. I even, half-jokingly, mentioned fly agaric.

'Fly what?'

'Fly agaric, Sares. It's an extraordinary fungus. You know – the classic red toadstool with white spots you see in children's books, usually with a pixie on top.'

'And...?'

'It's got all sorts of euphoric properties and the reindeer adore it. The Sàmi reindeer herders only have to scatter a few dried fragments on the snow to draw the reindeer in and dope them up, all ready for herding. It's a very neat trick.'

'Yes, but–' She was evidently going to point out that we weren't in Lapland.

'And guess what, Sares?' I interrupted enthusiastically. 'You can collect the reindeers' urine and drink it and it has just the same effect on us!'

She stared at me pityingly, not overly impressed by this outstanding piece of trivia. 'Charming!' She paused, then went on in a mock-serious tone: 'Well, I hate to pick holes in your fabulous list, but for a start, lemmings are in short supply. And on top of that, there are no eggs, frogs or magic mushrooms to be had.' She burst out laughing. 'OK, I'm going to be helpful now. Lichen you can harvest from nearby ridges. And how about haylage? Jimmy makes pretty good haylage.'

Jimmy Forster, Sares's father, ran Bold Cove, a high-welfare farm at Port Howard along the steep coastal ridges of the Falkland Sound. His grass-fed beef cattle were renowned for their temperament and excellent quality. This was the first time I had heard of anyone making haylage on the islands.

'Does he? Trust him! Can you persuade him to part with some for a good cause? Tell him I'll find a nice big set of antlers for his wall.' I paused. 'Then there's cattle nuts, I'll take a sack of those. What else, what else? What would tempt an animal from the Arctic Circle, what would be irresistible?'

'The comforting embrace of a polar bear?' She then made an unlikely suggestion. 'Hey, JoJoe, here's a thought. How about beet?'

'Beetroot? No way.'

'No! Sugar beet. Pat Witney imports dried sugar beet for his racehorse. I'm sure he'll let you have a few kilos.'

'Really?' I was sceptical. 'I don't think sugar beet exactly litters the Arctic tundra, Sares. They won't eat something they have no knowledge of. Like sheep. Surround them with unfamiliar feed and they'd rather starve to death than eat it.'

'It was only a suggestion. Anyway, sheep aren't exactly the brightest. They're always committing suicide.'

'Yes, you're right. I'm being unnecessarily negative. Why not? Let's give it a go. Nothing to lose, everything to gain.'

A FINGER IN THE DYKE

A few days later I touched down on the grass landing strip at Hill Cove. Peter Nightingale hefted my gear and took me to his neat airy house on the fringe of the pleasantly open village, brisk with a sea breeze.

Peter and Shelley were the farmers of West Lagoons and had a good reputation for their MPMs: Multi-purpose Merinos. By careful breeding and selection of their Merino flock, they had achieved some of the finest low-micron wool on the islands, perfect for the richly rewarding Italian suit market rather than the cheap dumping ground of house insulation and carpets. They were diligent farmers and excellent hosts, and I felt genuinely sorry for them. The reindeer had been a project they had seized on with enthusiasm, but it had become an embarrassing millstone. Peter was as keen as me to catch the herd and move them off his land.

In the evening Peter and I sat down in the living room with a beer, and I explained that no fault lay at their door. It had simply gone wrong. Having explored every inch of Rapid Point's dismal terrain and gleaned what I could from the relevant literature, I was able to see all the pieces of the puzzle.

In truth, I didn't much take to Rapid Point. It was partly instinctive and partly factual. It had the feel of sour land, perhaps too much poisoned by centuries of windblown brine, too much leached of nutrients by drenchings of rain. There were no rocky outcrops to speak of, and so no lichen and limited shelter. There was no decent permanent water, only brackish puddles and bogs. No trees to crop, of course, as the islands have a virtually treeless landscape. No great abundance or diversity of grasses, sedges or mosses, partly the result of the herd necessarily being confined by a deer fence and overgrazing the land. On top of that, the previous poor summer had been followed by an exceptionally severe winter, impeding feed regeneration so that the animals lacked an insulating layer of fat and burned off extra calories just keeping warm. And I had collected faecal samples on my last visit to find that the reindeer were riddled with parasitic worms picked up from the cattle, the typical last calling card prior to death. Parasites are great opportunists and take advantage of poor nutritional status and failing immune systems. When the doors of the warehouse fall open, they pour in like looters and raid what's left.

'Then there's the Falklands Factor,' added Peter, a fit, lean man with intense freckles and a receding hairline of gingery-grey hair. His face took no tan and had been reddened by the wind.

The Falklands Factor was the catch-all for those immutable difficulties encountered living on the edge of feasible existence where nature still holds the reins. It was really a combination of climate, topography and the ever-prevailing curse of mineral deficiency. For herbivores, there is no corner shop. Everything they need for growth, life and reproduction has to come out of the ground.

Peter outlined his plan. He had a set of cattle hurdles: rigid, connectable, six-foot high, tubular fence sections that could be assembled into any configuration. Along with the equally high deer fence, the idea was to shape a bottlenecked capture pen with a wide tapering mouth to channel the reindeer and drive them in, very much the same principle as a lobster pot, but for quadrupeds not decapods.

A good plan, but with one major stumbling block. 'The only trouble is, they don't drive. They have this powerful escape reflex. We found that out all too well last year. But I'm afraid that's for you to work out, Joe, that's your job.'

'What about sheepdogs?'

Peter raised his eyebrows. 'Too fast for dogs. And I've let them out from behind the deer fence so they can find more food. They'd run for miles.'

'They're no longer fenced in? You do know they're migratory?'

'Yes. They could run all the way to Port Howard if they wanted to, but they don't. They hang around by the deer fence. I had to do it, but you're right,' he went on, noting my pained expression, 'we might just see their backsides disappearing over the horizon. It's not going to be easy.'

'Sure, I understand.' Freeing them from Rapid Point had been a sensible precaution considering they seemed to be dropping like flies. 'OK, Peter, we just have to try. Once we're all set up, I'll go and stay with them. I've got my tent and sleeping bag and some essential provisions. I'll do my best to make them trust me. Then I'll play it by ear.' I took a determined swig of beer.

All the next day we toiled hard at Rapid Point, dragging and juggling twenty-six giant hurdles into the beginnings of a trap, but the herd had moved across the boggy flats to the distant slopes of Channel Hill, a ridge well over a mile away. This was a worrying complication. The image of receding backsides loomed strong in my mind.

Three times a day I crossed over and fed them, not only to habituate them to my presence, but also to make them think of me as the candy man. It was a good opportunity to study my quarry. The tastes of reindeer, lemmings notwithstanding, are clearly very specific. We knew, for example, that they wouldn't eat sheep nuts, but cattle nuts – little brown pellets of protein and fibre – were a familiar feed from their days on the government farm, and if I placed my yellow bucket down and walked away, the reindeer tucked in. The haylage, deliciously fragrant and reminiscent of sports days and new-mown meadows, was spurned, though there was nothing wrong with it and Peter's cattle demolished it with gusto. Starving, and yet fussy: it seemed reindeer were the herbivore equivalent of cats.

All the same, I was beguiled. Such gentle creatures, with long horsey faces and cow-like eyes, creamy-grey pelts tinged with chocolate – now sadly bedraggled and moth-eaten – and absurdly disproportionate side-plate hooves. They were mostly cows, with one mature stag and one back-up yearling stag: a reasonably balanced herd. Only a few stick-like antlers remained after their annual shedding and a couple of the cows were bagging up with milk, a sure sign they were on the brink of calving.

And yet for all this, it was a struggle to get them to trust me. Their escape reflex, genetically embedded for fleeing the sudden onrush of the wolf, was well developed. A sudden move on my part, a flick of the hand or a hasty crouch, and they vanished, as if by sleight of hoof, and then moments later there they would be in the distance, heads back down and grazing as if nothing had happened. This was not fright, but pure tactical flight, putting a quick safe distance between the herd and the enemy. Day by day I lured them closer to the deer fence, and day by day they began to look at me with more benevolent recognition. But I still couldn't get near them. As far as they were concerned, I was a potential predator.

Next, I broke out the molassed sugar beet. The trouble with molassed sugar beet, or perhaps its beauty, is that it needs soaking overnight, whereupon, like a biblical miracle, it expands to five times its original volume. Otherwise, it is inedible. I took water from the broad freshwater bog and worked the miracle overnight, then offered up the product for breakfast. I wasn't too optimistic.

There was a moment of hesitation, a lack of recognition but definite curiosity. The lead cow, in tatty coat and half-shed antlers, leaned into the bucket and sniffed its contents, then her prehensile lip muzzled into the dark brown mash. Suddenly she was wolfing it down and, seeing her approval of the novel taste, the other reindeer moved in and mobbed her. They tossed the bucket around, boxing for space with their muzzles and remaining antlers, scattering the mash and hoovering it up. They adored it.

Astounding. I had my fly agaric after all. Thank you, Sarah Bowles.

The following day I laid down trails of sugar-beet mash leading towards the fledgling capture pen. During the night it vanished, and the herd lingered around. The worrying complication had been laid to rest. We had finally succeeded in enticing them back in from the distant hill; an embryonic trust was growing.

Four days in, and the capture pen was only half assembled. The received wisdom from the herders in Alaska was that the whole cumbersome affair had to be shrouded in burlap – and we had yet to do this task of giant tailoring. Without the burlap, reindeer see a horizon, an escape route, and can attempt to climb out. The great flared mouth of the pen was set and open, ready for the day when we would try to drive or lure them in, and we had yet to fit a gate to the gap in the deer fence we had opened so that we could move back and forth.

I laced the ground inside the pen with my latest brew of sugar beet, and crawled into my flimsy orange tent, alone but more than happy to lie there listening to the whisper of the breeze and the soft hiss of the surf on the shingle. Weary from the day's labours, my loyal yellow bucket of expanding sugar beet beside me, I soon slid into a deep sleep.

I woke to the insipid light of early morning and reluctantly dragged myself out of the cosy warmth of my sleeping bag. The inside of the tent was slick with condensation, and my clothes felt damp and sticky with salt and perspiration. Outside, the sea mists had coated the ground with a heavy dew which glowed pale in the low, feeble sunshine. Soon it would be a glorious day, but for now I felt cold, stiff and dirty. I straightened up outside the tent, rubbed my bleary eyes and stretched into the sky, then reached down, soggy headed, to pull on a heavy fleece. The narcotic murmurings of dawn were ruptured by a distinct, long and melodious burp.

There they were, the whole herd, lying down behind the tent, chewing the cud. One by one they stood and watched me with their dark, glassy eyes, expectant and trusting. Outwardly, I must have looked as if I'd been turned to stone, but my mind was rushing with colliding possibilities. Slowly, ever so slowly, my own eyes fixed on theirs, I crouched down and fumbled blindly for the yellow bucket, then walked, half turning to the herd, towards the entrance of the trap, sprinkling my offerings of sugar beet as I went.

This was my Pied Piper moment. They came, nuzzling the ground for the fragments, and followed me in, every single one of them. I scattered the remaining contents of the bucket and backed away. My heart was pounding with adrenaline because this was the event, the key event we had been planning for – but not yet. We weren't ready. No burlap, the flared entrance unsecured, the gap in the deer fence still very much a gap, and absolutely no means of capture. What was I doing? This was no trap; this was more of an agricultural art installation.

Yet the reindeer looked relaxed. Then, to my utter amazement, having devoured the beet, each one lay down, taking their cue from the leader, and, eyes half closed in contentment, began once more to chew the cud.

It was an opportunity too good to miss. I had to gamble.

I crept round to the gaping defect of the entrance and with painstakingly slow tugs pulled the heavy hurdles across until they met, forensically observing every animal for a reaction. But there were only idle glances as their jaws ground rhythmically in almost orchestral unison and they savoured the flow of tasty juices. I had the pleasant dawning realisation that I was no longer seen as a potential predator. I was still not their master, but at least for now I was an adopted friend of the herd.

There was one other major defect. I stood in the gap in the deer fence, a pathetically ineffectual obstruction, trying to look big and impassable yet totally unsure of my next move. I had them. But then again, I really didn't.

The Land Rover was alongside the fence just a few feet away. I sidled towards it, squinting sideways for reaction, released the handbrake and rolled it back so that it was closer, then very quietly emptied the vehicle of everything it had to offer: spare tyre, plastic containers, assorted clothing and tool box. Item by item, using the spare tyre as the centrepiece, I built the soundest barrier I could devise, no easy task in slow motion and near-total silence. The result looked farcical, but it was the best I could do. I fetched some cattle nuts, my supply of soaked sugar beet having been exhausted, and cast handfuls into the pen like heavy confetti. I wanted the reindeer to feel as if they had been trapped in a sweet shop, which is no trap at all.

Then I reached for the 2-metre VHF radio under the dash and stretched the coiled cable of the handset almost to snapping point so that I could still stand in the gap. The day was yet young.

I pressed the side button. 'Joe Hollins on Rapid Point, Joe Hollins on Rapid Point, can anyone hear me? Over.'

The Atlantic sighed back across the airways. Nothing.

'It's Joe Hollins, Joe Hollins calling, is there anyone out there? Over.'

The receiver burst into life, boomingly clear. 'Hello, Joe Hollins, what are you doing on Rapid Point? Over.' It was David Poll-Evans on the wildlife haven of Saunders Island, visible across the water. He was sounding amused and curious. David was an early riser and liked to listen to the traffic on the 2-metre radio, a staple of communication on the islands before the rise of the mobile phone. He was a stoutly built man with a matching sense of humour, drily concealed beneath a deadpan face. I had the feeling he either took to you or didn't with no shades of grey in between, but I'd had the good fortune to operate successfully on a newborn calf of his, removing a grossly traumatised eyeball, and it had cemented our friendship. I enjoyed his company enormously.

'Hi David. It sounds like you're the only one awake.' I quickly explained about the reindeer and my predicament. 'Could you telephone Peter Nightingale and tell him to get out here as soon as possible?'

'So... you're standing in a gap in this trap that isn't a trap with a spare tyre and a herd of reindeer?' The speaker vibrated with his deep belly laughs. 'You're like that little boy with his finger in the hole.'

'Dyke, David. It was a dyke.'

'Oh - a dyke! What was his name?'

'Hans, David, his name was Hans. Yes, I'm like Hans with his finger in the dyke.' I was trying not to laugh, but David's guffaws were infectious. 'Can you help me?'

'Of course,' he replied, suddenly serious. 'Just hang on there and I'll give him a call.' Then, in a final fit of laughter, he added: 'Don't go anywhere, Hans! Over and out.'

Moments later he radioed back. 'I've got hold of Peter. It's a Sunday morning of course and he's entertaining some councillor. But he said he'd be out as soon as possible. I guess it takes a while to get there.'

'At least an hour.'

'Well, keep that finger in the... er... dyke.' More belly laughs. 'No doubt I'll hear how it all goes. Good luck. Over and out.'

In light of the previous mob-handed capture attempt and the fact that the reindeer were now habituated to our company, Peter and I had already agreed that no other assistance would be called upon as strangers might spook our sensitive animals. And Peter had exactly the right calm and sensitive disposition for the task. I felt we made the perfect team.

It was four achingly long hours before I saw Peter weaving his way along the only track through the peat bogs in a small tractor towing a flatbed trailer. A tractor is a powerful and dependable beast, and not the fastest of travellers, but he had thought it through. If we managed to catch the herd, the tractor and trailer would be the only way to get them out of there without getting bogged down, which would spell an ignoble end to our worthy endeavours.

Peter pulled up and leaped out of the cab. 'Wow. We really have them.' He patted me on the back. 'Well done, Joe. Sorry about the delay but I came as soon as I could.' He grabbed a gate from the trailer and quickly secured the gap. I was free.

'Where's the livestock trailer, Peter?' I asked, mystified, stretching my limbs.

'Aha!' He pushed his sunglasses back on the bridge of his nose and tapped the side of his head. 'We're going to build one.'

The next few hours were a lesson in Falkland ingenuity.

First, we cloaked the whole capture pen with burlap, securing it top and bottom with strands of unravelled rope. Our Alaskan

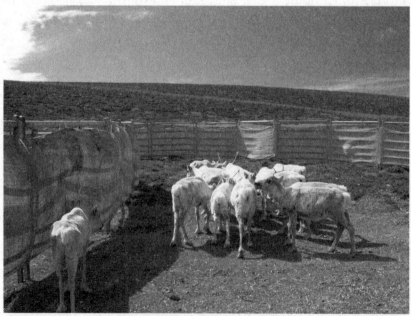

The herd of depleted reindeer inside our makeshift
pen, awaiting transfer to Albemarle

herder friends would have been proud. Then we shrank the pen, hurdle by hurdle, to reduce the interior area. This we did with minimal noise and movement, closely observing the animals for signs of stress or rising panic and allowing them to settle down each time. Occasionally I threw in handfuls of nuts or sugar-beet mash to keep them occupied.

We then constructed the livestock trailer using six of the released hurdles which we pinned together and lashed onto the flatbed with trailer straps. The whole assemblage was reinforced with wire salvaged from a nearby disused fence, chocks of drift-wood from the beach nailed onto the wooden flatbed, and zigzags of rope. I clambered over the cage-like structure performing surgery: sewing on overlapping sheets of burlap with more lengths of fencing wire, certainly the coarsest suture material I had ever used, until it was completely covered bar the rear. A hurdle was left to hinge as a loading gate, and a divider inserted to stop the reindeer bunching on the bumpy journey to Hill Cove. We shrank the capture pen further, and used a pallet to construct a ramp to marry up with the rear of the trailer. Finally, we were ready for the tricky bit: loading the reindeer without losing them.

Peter grabbed the lead cow and pulled her up the ramp, securing her in the trailer pen as bait. Together we pulled in the sides of the capture pen, hinging in the hurdles until they folded onto themselves, so that the pen became small and tight, and the herd compressed. I gently tried to usher them forward. They milled around, bumping into each other and occasionally tapping their hooves on the wooden ramp, becoming alarmed by the unfamiliar feel and the clacking sound. I sensed their rising panic. One animal reared up and tried to climb over the side of the ramp, the weak point in our construction. She could see out; she could sense freedom. My heart was in my mouth. If one went, they'd all go, and I'd never gain their trust again. This was the defining moment: win or lose, now or never. I grabbed her hind leg and pulled her down, then we both threw ourselves against the herd, arms spread wide. There was a clatter of feet and a surge. They were in.

Peter and I looked at each other in total disbelief, beaming from ear to ear. We wired up the rear gate, covered it in burlap, and surveyed our captives, peering through the mesh of the fabric into the dimly lit interior. The reindeer stood placidly awaiting the next act. They had finally submitted.

'Right,' said Peter. 'Let's get out of here or we'll end up thigh deep in a bog.' The sun was sinking, and the light beginning to dim.

For the next two hours, while I shadowed him in the Land Rover, Peter negotiated the tractor and trailer across the peat and then along the dirt road to Hill Cove. In my headlights, our burlapped monstrosity flapped, wobbled and shook like a tumbrel on the way to the guillotine, but it served its purpose well. It held together.

Hill Cove is no more than a straggle of fenced white houses with red and green tin roofs, lapped by the ocean and separated by liberal carpets of grass. We pulled up at the communal wool-shed, strategically positioned at one end of the broad, central track, and carefully offloaded the reindeer into the slatted sheep pens. It was after midnight, Monday morning. It had been the longest of days. Back at Peter's house, over mugs of tea, I debated phoning Vic and telling him the good news.

'Yes, go on. Wake the bugger up, he won't mind,' urged Peter. 'Phone's over there.'

I listened to the ringing tone at the other end in Stanley, wondering if Vic would explode.

'Yup.' Vets are used to being disturbed at ridiculous hours.

'Hi Vic, it's Joe.'

'Whadya want?' His voice was thick with sleep.

'I have them, Vic. I have the herd. Peter and I caught them, and we've brought them in to Hill Cove and put them in the woolshed to settle overnight. Sorry about the late call but we've only just come in. Thought you'd like to know.'

He did explode - with delight. 'What? The whole herd? You have them? The whole herd?' It was very rare that Vic threw me a compliment, but I knew deep down he was deeply troubled by the potential scandal of the lost reindeer, and he dropped his guard. 'Joe, you beauty. That's bloody wonderful. That's made my week.'

'What do you want me to do, Vic? Shall I come back to Stanley?'

'Bloody hell, no. Stay - stay as long as you need. Finish the job. Organise a cattle truck first thing and get them down to Cape Meredith. Don't come back until it's done. And Joe - fantastic. Now go get some sleep.' High praise indeed from the laconic Vic.

Peter drained his tea and put down his mug with exhausted finality. 'So, what's the plan?'

'I need to organise a cattle truck. Who do we ask, Peter?'

'Leon Marsh. He'll help us out. Now, I don't know about you, but I'm knackered. Time to get some shut-eye.'

The next morning brought fresh complications. Peter had already been out to check the reindeer. Shelley, a handsome, practical woman, was standing in the living room cradling a small, sleek, glossy bundle, her head bowed attentively as she rocked it from side to side. Two stunningly large, dark, shiny orbs looked out from the crook of her elbow. It was a calf, fresh to the world and one of the most beautiful newborns I have ever laid eyes upon. I was once again struck by the purity of innocence that radiates from any newborn, and this creature was Bambi by the shedload.

'She's premature and has hypothermia,' Shelley said. 'Probably born just after you got in. The mother is a maiden cow and shows no interest. All legs!' she added with a grin, showing me the calf's underside.

'I was afraid of this,' I said. 'I don't think it'll be the last. Several are about to pop.' Then, genuinely awed, stroking the silky head: 'God, Shelley, she's lovely.'

'We'll do our best to hand rear her. We've done enough orphan lambs in the past. But I don't know – she's so weak. She needs the beastings.'

Beastings is the first milk, a custard-like substance more technically known as colostrum. It is Mother Nature's great gift, an ingenious, life-preserving elixir, rich in protective antibodies, minerals and nutrition, all designed to protect a precious new life propelled from the protective haven of the womb into a filthy, chilly, germ-laden world. Without colostrum, a newborn tends to die, overwhelmed by some everyday microbe.

I went over to the woolshed and with Peter restraining the mother, milked off as much beastings as I could. But after ten days of diligent bottle feeding, and despite Shelley's dedicated and tender loving care, the pretty little calf broke our hearts and succumbed to a fatal dysentery.

Fortunately, though, she wasn't the only new arrival – more were on the way.

TRANSLOCATION

West Falkland is larger than you might think. From Hill Cove on the northern tip to Cape Meredith on the southern tip is a grinding, hundred-mile trek through rolling hills and craggy peaks on dicey gravel roads. After hours of careful driving, Leon Marsh's bright-orange cattle truck crested a ridge north of Port Stephens and pulled over for a rest. Peter and I were following in a car. We were a tiny travelling circus.

The day had begun in piercing, early morning sunlight, catching the village gorse in full flower, dazzling yellow and fragrant. Now the land was coated in a gentle haze, and beyond to the south lay inlet after inlet, separated by bulging hills of cinnamon brown mottled by black stains of peat and grey crusts of rock. Somewhere deep in the haze, secreted beyond the maze of land and sea, down a long, sinuous, dead-end track, lay the sheep farm Albemarle, encompassing Cape Meredith and the Three Crowns.

Peter climbed up the slatted aluminium sides of the cattle truck and checked our wards. 'Uh-uhh!' He turned his head with a look of resignation. 'We have another baby.' I quickly joined him. Then, more happily: 'Oh but look – he's standing and suckling his mum. And she's cooing to him. Obviously not a first timer.'

We lowered ourselves down inside and partitioned her off. Reindeer cows would normally hide away to calve, only to re-join the herd after a couple of days once the calf is strong and able to look out for itself. This enforced confinement, to her a public spectacle, must have felt like a gross violation of her basic instincts, and yet she looked to be coping remarkably well.

THE SHEPHERD'S SHANTY

Leon Berntsen leaned against the heavy tread on the rear tyre of his tractor and carefully rolled a cigarette, fingers adept at securing the loose tobacco in the wind. He was wearing a brown leather deerstalker, ears buttoned up, not a Sherlockian affectation but a hugely practical hat for the buffeting, ear-aching winds of the islands.

Before us a blue-black sea crashed against a great arc of crumbling, biscuit-coloured cliff, and above, beyond the deer fence along the top of a steep, grassy flank, stood the splendid Three Crowns, three huge and perfectly aligned sentinels of rock, fragmented remains of a higher plateau that looked more like ruined castle keeps or giant decayed teeth than royal headwear.

There was no pediment at the base of the cliffs, no beach to pacify the waves, just pure, eternal, thrashing ocean.

'I lost a bullock over there once,' he said, having lit his rollie. 'It panicked and ran full gallop over the edge. Hit the water like a bomb.'

'Killed it, I suppose.'

'No – surprisingly.'

'Oh! Can cattle swim?'

He grunted. 'Barely.'

'What did you do?'

'What could I do?' he replied with emphasis. 'I put it out of its misery. I shot it.'

It conjured up a dramatic image, Leon with his rifle at the cliff edge, legs apart to steady his aim, the barrel angled sharply down past his feet and into the sea, the bullock bellowing madly as it floundered and choked in the surf. Almost an oil painting.

The tractor was hitched to a trailer of dark-green planking, extended with chipboard panels and covered over according to prior instructions from Peter. On the side of his ramshackle creation Leon had proudly tacked a large piece of white card that said quite simply in tall black capitals: 'REINDEER TRUCK'. Inside, the reindeer waited patiently with an occasional tapping of hooves, sensing freedom and a new beginning.

It had been a long trip up from the Albemarle house, across the ubiquitous peat bogs, around the head of a deep inlet called Kit's Cove where Leon told me they once landed the bottles of acetylene and loaded them onto mules to feed the beacon on Cape Meredith, then up and over drier slopes to a raised coastline. A perfect green and white shepherd's shanty with enclosed sheepdog pens squatted in a shallow vale where a gurgling stream, deeply slotted into the peat, ran down to the cliff. The deer fence stretched away from us in both directions.

I hadn't had a chance to meet Leon Berntsen before the previous night, when our travelling circus had pulled up in his yard. Ingeniously constructed from the remains of the Port Albemarle sealing station, his farmhouse was spacious and homely, with views out across a bay to the Arch Islands. We had turned the reindeer out into the woolshed and fed them with buckets of lichen, which they gorged on with great happiness. The new mother and calf had been given the privacy of their own pen and had bonded well. Leaning on the wooden rails watching that unbreakable union develop gave us the greatest of pleasures. Then we had gone indoors to feed ourselves on a sumptuous meal laid on by Pam, Leon's wife. The frenetic pace of the last few days was over. I felt myself melt in the cheery warmth, relieved of my responsibilities and the spectre of failure. Beer was drunk.

A former police officer, Leon came across as a reserved man, brief and considered in his speech. It became rapidly apparent to me, though, that beneath that controlled, slightly serious exterior lay a very decent, capable man, and his small leakages of gentle humour made me warm to him immediately.

'So... what do you think?' he asked now.

'What do I think?' I took in the seascape, the long ribbon of cliff, the Three Crowns, the vista. I was overwhelmed by its raw beauty. 'Leon... it's magnificent.'

'I've been waiting for this so long,' he stated distantly. 'I built the reindeer fence a couple of years ago. It's a headland of about fifteen hundred acres, the same as Rapid Point. That's about the only similarity. Over there, they have access to a long sandy beach, then the coastline sweeps round into the entrance of a big bay, Port Stephens - full of islands - then back up into Kit's Cove.'

'Where's Cape Meredith?'

He turned and pointed in the other direction to where the cliffs curved and disappeared behind a high bluff. 'Some geologists came here once and got very excited. Said the Cape had fragments of the Earth's mantle. Rare apparently. Kept chipping away at the cliffs with their hammers.'

This was an ancient world, right on the edge of existence.

Leon turned to Pam, standing silently nearby, and with an unusual thrill of excitement in his voice said, 'Well, Pam - it's time. Let's do it.'

He backed the trailer through the opening in the deer fence, snugged its rear against a bank and dropped the tailgate. We waited on tenterhooks.

They came, at first cautiously, their lustrous eyes taking in their new home, then in a rush, stopping a few metres from the trailer and looking back with a hint of suspicion. The newly calved cow moved apart from the herd, her lanky-legged baby trotting happily beside her before thrusting underneath to suckle. The rest relaxed and put their heads down to graze.

It was a tatty-looking herd and would win no prizes, but I couldn't help feeling just a little triumphant pride. This was completion. 'Look at that, Leon – they're going to be just fine. You have your reindeer at last.'

He was staring at the herd. 'Yes – my reindeer,' he whispered with mild disbelief. He turned to me with watery eyes. Probably just the biting wind. 'Thank you, Joe.'

For a while we watched the herd settle in, then Leon stirred. 'Come,' he said. 'I've something to show you.'

Shepherds' shanties, built in the days before the combustion engine provided the luxury of whizzing the sheep hands back to home fires every evening, speckle the remoter parts of the Falkland landscape and are in themselves an architectural art form, each slightly varied in colour, shape, dog pens and wall panelling, according to the whims of the men who constructed them. Leon's was outstanding.

Such was his love of heritage that he had completely restored his shanty, with fastidious care and attention to detail: exterior walls dazzling white, two wood-framed, six-paned windows and door all stained moss green, and a new, pea-green corrugated-iron roof pierced by a central stone chimney. Leon explained how the shepherds would be cut off, sometimes for days, by the weather or have a grand muster to undertake at the time of shearing or need to watch over and attend to the ewes at lambing, and the shanty was their shelter and their haven.

'And they left behind something special which I've tried to preserve.' He took me through the bunk room into the sitting area. The walls and ceiling were boarded in deeply honeyed tongue-and-groove pine, but one whole wall had in effect been wallpapered, with wallpaper of a fascinating kind: pages from magazines dated 1927 and 1928, including *Tatler*, *All Sports Weekly* and the *Illustrated Sporting and Dramatic News*. There were square-rigger sailing ships and yachting regattas alongside dancers with bouffant dresses from the latest production of *The Moulin Rouge* at the Tivoli, and a fivesome of flappers called The Rough House Rosie Company under the headline: 'Some Bright Stars from the Flickers in the USA'. There were posed profiles of shining racehorses, and hunting scenes of riders clearing fences; then, in total contrast, 'Ranching in Patagonia' with gauchos on horseback lassoing cattle, far closer to the Falklands than the sport of kings. There were rowers, 'Christs Crew: Winners of the Cambridge Clinker Fours', rubbing shoulders with a moorland scene of a strapping lady in plus fours reaching a gauntleted fist into the sky to receive a huge Golden Eagle, 'The Greatest of Our Birds of Prey'. Extraordinary 'Feats of Strength and Skill' were being performed by a troupe of lithe 'German Girl Gymnasts' at the Coliseum, tumbling across a field spread-eagled in giant spinning wheels known

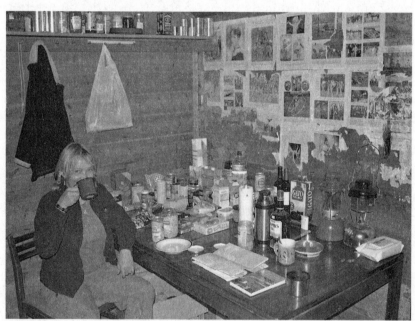

Teeny Lucy and our Old Year's Night feast inside
the shepherd's shanty at Three Crowns

as Rhönrads, while above, a po-faced Miss Richmond in full hunting garb, the 'well known breeder of deerhounds' with 'an establishment at Henley-on-Thames', holds the reins of her horse as she is mobbed by a dozen of her shaggy 'friendly giants'. More plus fours and high woollen socks on a smartly dressed country gentleman, member of 'Lord Dunraven's fishing party' in Ireland, wearing tweed cap, heavy jacket and watch chain as, with the slightest of smiles, he dangles a large plump salmon; then just below, three actresses lean against tall park railings backed by ghostly silhouettes of trees to illustrate 'Nöel Coward wit in *This Year of Grace*' at the London Pavilion. And one notice, perhaps a lasting tease by a Scottish shepherd, for a football clash: 'Scotland's Soccer Victory: England Outplayed. The Association football match between England and Scotland played before a vast crowd at Wembley Stadium was won by the latter by five goals to one – and then some, as the Americans would say'. As they might, but probably not about soccer. It was a time capsule, a glimpse into the thoughts, yearnings and aspirations of 1920s Falkland shepherds sitting out storms and chilly nights in far-flung isolation.

'Leon, it's a treasure trove.' I pored over the pictures and articles of the prosperous and jubilant Roaring Twenties, post the-war-to-end-all-wars, and as yet blind to the imminence of fascism, the Great Depression and yet another devastating world war. 'Do you think this is what they missed and that's why they pasted them up there, or just something to brighten up their lives and distract them from their harsh existence?'

'Who knows? The islands were in the hands of the wool barons then, but these are scenes from lives the average shepherd could never lead.'

Of course. I got it. This was escapism, something to keep the imagination alive, and the belief in greater things.

'Anyway, Joe, if you ever want a break, come and stay here. Now – let's go home and eat.'

That night I slept like a dead man and awoke, utterly refreshed, to the soothing, primal sounds of wind and sea. It had been ten tiring – though most rewarding – days since leaving Stanley, and this was to be my last full day before flying back. Over tea and toast Leon regaled me with stories of times past: of hardy landsmen, failed sealing enterprises, and the Argentinian invasion. I could have listened to him all day, but I had a personal agendum to fulfil. Leon was my co-conspirator – also enthusiastic about the Cape Meredith beacon, although perhaps not quite to the point of obsession, as I was.

'It's a work of genius,' he explained. 'A miracle of engineering. And it must be about the only one left in situ and completely intact. No vandals or trophy hunters out here.' He laughed his rare laugh, then leaned forward over the toast crumbs. 'It has a sun valve.'

'What on earth is a sun valve?' The name was enticing.

'You've not heard of it? Well, you'll be looking at a device that earned the inventor a Nobel Prize. You won't miss it – if you don't get lost on the way that is. Oh, and mind the sea lions.'

Sea lions on land are like bad-tempered muggers. 'Where are they?'

'Just as you approach the beacon there is a large colony hauled up from the cove. You have to pass through them, but just check the tussac as you go. They shelter in the grass and if you cut off their path to the sea, before you know it, you'll be on the ground kissing fishy whiskers with a chunk out of your leg.'

THE GREAT ILLUMINATOR

I didn't know what to expect. But what I found was a glorious thing.

I left the Land Rover where the terrain became impassable and ventured forward on foot. The muggers were there, lurking in the tussac, bewhiskered and growly, barking out their disapproval as I trespassed through their realm. Among them, a gang of striated caracaras, birds of prey with a cheeky attitude, strutted about, sharp-eyed, intent on some form of avian mischief. Below, a tumble of sea-chewed boulders led down to a melancholy cove of foaming surf. An ancient, weary cliff loomed beyond, its base stained black and pounded ceaselessly by a frantic disarray of Atlantic rollers. I could feel Cape Meredith's primeval origins, its timelessness, its complete indifference to humankind. And yet humankind was not indifferent to Cape Meredith. On the very tip of the cape stood an icon to scientific achievement: the extraordinary inventor Gustaf Dalén's beacon and his still glittering, enigmatic sun valve.

The beacon stood defiantly in the bullying wind, illuminated by the sharp austral summer sunshine against the spuming ocean, which stretched away with nothing to impede it until the great white continent of Antarctica.

It was raised aloft on a grey, rust-streaked galvanised chamber, a sort of trapezoid coffin designed both to contain the acetylene cylinders and act as a tall pedestal. On top of this, a small, railed walkway no larger than a family dining table encircled a sturdy, flat-topped, four-legged iron stool held together with rivets the size of hazelnuts. Crowning this brute structure, raised into the heavens like an ascending deity and no larger than a fat keg of beer, sat the lantern, a perfect union of practicality and aesthetics. Mostly it was crystal, an outer protective cylinder of thick glass embracing the even thicker, flawlessly curved, heavily ridged

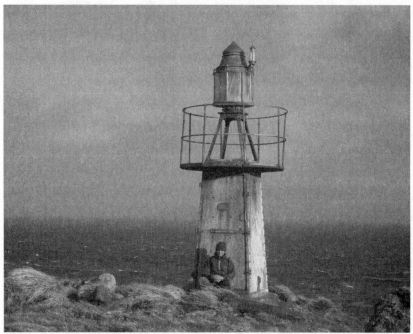

At the Cape Meredith beacon

lenses for intensifying the bright white light of the acetylene flame within. All was held together by the armour of a pleasingly contoured brass casing with a vented conical roof, now burnished to bronze and gleaming in the sunlight with highlights of verdigris.

And then there was a work of art, a shining jewel. Held away from the conical roof by an elegant bracket to avoid all shadow, and fed by two spiralling brass tubes, was a small device that reeked of intelligent design: the sun valve. Vertical strips of black and gold flashed brilliantly in a tapering glass tube of infinite purity, capped with a miniature Pickelhaube, a Bismarckian spiked helmet. Catching sight of this whimsical flourish, I couldn't help but smile and nod my approval.

The sun valve was so transformative for navigation at sea – and therefore so lifesaving – that it earned Dalén the Nobel Prize in physics, awarded just a few weeks after he destroyed his eyes in an acetylene explosion trying to perfect his creation. Such cruel irony, to lose his vision inventing devices that could be seen. Pictures of Dalén reveal a handsome man with high cheekbones, a receding hairline and a vigorous moustache, though in his later years he took on a slightly eerie appearance by concealing his damaged eyes behind dark goggles.

I was surprised to see a warm, familiar, friendly acronym pressed into the brass casing of the beacon: AGA, which stood for Aktiebolaget Gas Accumulator. This Swedish company, of which Dalén was chief engineer, specialised in acetylene gas, which burns with a dazzling white light and was therefore superior to other fuels in terms of visibility. It was – and is – the very same company that went on to produce the AGA cooker, another Dalén invention considered quintessentially British farmhouse, yet solidly Swedish in origin. Astonishingly, he developed it after he was blinded when he realised the extent of his wife's burden in keeping the family fed. The AGA stove was more economical on coal and allowed a flexible approach to cooking.

Dalén's constant drive was economy. Acetylene had a disadvantage: it was hugely expensive and the continuous burning of the gas in lighthouses and beacons greatly limited its application. The beautiful sun valve was a set of bimetallic strips that distorted in the sun to close a valve and shut off the gas during daylight. This and other refinements – such as the Dalén Flasher, a gas regulator that caused the flame to burn intermittently and thus more conspicuously – reduced gas consumption by 94 per cent and slashed the cost of navigation lights. Now the essence of the man's genius stood before me on an ancient headland in the deep South Atlantic. No battery, no silicon chip, no algorithm, just pure applied physics. Bravo, Gustaf.

On the way back to Albemarle I diverted up the track to the Three Crowns to check on the reindeer, elated by my day of discovery and confident of our total success. One was missing.

I searched and searched until the light faded and I could search no more. The next morning, Leon, knowing well the lie of his land, soon located her body in the deep-cut stream that flowed to the cliff edge. Too weak to climb out, she had succumbed to the chill of the water.

I was deflated. No sooner had the numbers gone up than they had come down again. I had been foolishly overconfident of success and flush from my visit to the beacon. Suddenly, it seemed to me that the whole project still hung in the balance.

RESURRECTION

The Christmas break rolled around – midsummer in the Falklands – and for once I was off-duty, so I decided to take Leon up on his offer to stay in the shepherd's shanty.

My long-suffering girlfriend Teeny Lucy was over for a visit from the UK and I wanted to treat her. I shipped my Land Rover Defender across Falkland Sound on the inter-island ferry and drove her down to Cape Meredith. We stocked the shanty with festive bounty: cardboard boxes crammed with calorific food and many clanking bottles. It was to be an austral equivalent of spending Hogmanay in a Scottish bothy, something she had desperately wanted to do.

In true Falkland style it poured with rain, drumming on the roof and saturating the bogs. The stream was soon in spate, rumbling past the shanty.

We didn't care. It was hugely atmospheric, and we were delightfully cut off.

On Old Year's Night, bellies full and pleasurably drunk, surrounded by the mellow pine walls glowing in the candle-light and the surreal audience of gentry, athletes and actors from the distant Roaring Twenties, we toasted the New Year through three time zones – the UK and then the two zones of the Falklands: 'Stanley time' for the town folk and, an hour later, 'Camp time' for the rural folk in *el campo*, as the still-used gaucho terminology has it.

Late in the morning on New Year's Day, the skies having finally rained themselves into grey exhaustion, we went in search of the reindeer. I was buzzing with anticipation. Leon had been deliberately restrained but there was a playful, teasing glint in his eye.

We criss-crossed the whole peninsula, climbed the Three Crowns, explored the beach, waded through the diddle-dee and fled from a sea lion that took the shortest available route

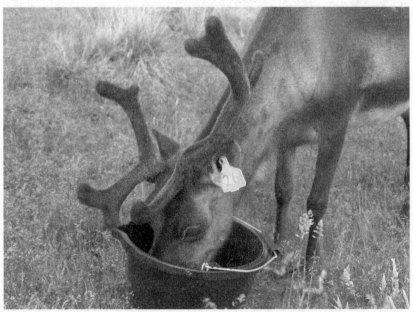

A rejuvenated reindeer feeding at Albemarle, New Year's Day

through our legs in an explosion of sand and tussac, but no reindeer were to be found. We sat wearily on the brow of the high hill that formed the central hub of the peninsula, our feet soggy and sore, and I stared morosely into the distance. The day was slipping away. Where were my lovely animals?

Teeny sat up with a jerk and pointed into the valley below. 'There! Look! What's that? Down there in the shadow. Is that them?'

We scrambled down the slope. I was astounded. The reindeer had transformed into Christmas card perfection. They had shed their tatty coats in favour of glossy pelts of cream, grey and brown, subtle camouflage that explained their melding into the landscape; their ribs had decent cover; and their heads were adorned with freshly sprouted antlers, wrapped in the finest velvet like a child's plush toy. And best of all, there were sixteen of them; four healthy young calves were trotting along at foot. My gorgeous reindeer were finally on the up.

A few years later, as planned, the South Georgia reindeer were successfully and humanely eradicated. To their surprise the authorities found that between the Barff herd and the Busen herd, they had to deal with just under 7,000 individuals. Now even the rats have been sent on their way, thanks to a huge rodent elimination programme that was probably enacted with less tender loving care, rats being far too clever for their own good. The whaling station of Grytviken, where Ernest Shackleton sleeps silently in his grave, stands conserved along with its abandoned steam whalers as a sprawling monument to humankind's indebtedness to our fellow creatures. Offshore, whales begin to spout once more, and the seals, penguins and albatross have reclaimed their stolen territory. The natural order of things is finally being restored.

DEATH OF A LIGHTHOUSE KEEPER

Not every story has a happy ending, of course, and this one is bittersweet. I had a deep, almost reverent respect for the quietly spoken Leon Berntsen, and he was the perfect man to tend and rear what I selfishly looked on as 'my' reindeer. I subsequently heard that he was intensely proud of them.

In a final act of acknowledgement for his kindness to me and his shared love of the animals I had rescued, I made him a member of the splendidly eccentric Association of Lighthouse Keepers. What, I thought, could be more fitting for a man who was caretaker of a Nobel Prize-winning beacon on the remotest of headlands. And I did so in the full knowledge that, to my very great sadness, he was dying of lung cancer.

He was buried in the peat of his beloved Albemarle, as is the custom of pioneering nations, ringed off from the livestock in the traditional way by a low, white picket fence. Each mourner went down to the grave, yarned to him, toasted him and anointed his mound with a generous tot of rum.

And the reindeer? What of the reindeer?

The reindeer are prospering. They now number some eighty head.

Sleep easy, my friend. Mission accomplished.

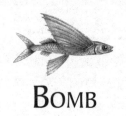

BOMB

Good morning, ladies and gentlemen, and welcome to Jamestown, St Helena Island, the emerald set in bronze. St Helena is the home of the oldest living land creature, the oldest Anglican church in the southern hemisphere, the death place of the great French emperor Napoleon, the refuge of many a poor soul during the slave trade, the home of the most isolated international airport in the world, and of course the spiritual home of RMS *St Helena*. Welcome.

Captain Adam Williams MBE after dropping anchor on
the final voyage of the RMS St Helena, 10 January 2018

IQUIQUE, ATACAMA COAST, NORTHERN CHILE

'Are you alone?'

'Yes... but it doesn't matter.' I leaned into the booth of the internet café, tired, dishevelled, and gritty from the desert.

'Are you sitting down?' continued the sympathetic voice 6,000 miles away. I could hear the bustle of the hospital corridors in the background.

'No.' It could only mean one thing. 'It's OK... just tell me.' I pinched the bridge of my nose to hold back the tears and sighed. 'He's dead, isn't he?'

Two months previously Phyl Rendell, the Falklands Director of Agriculture and Natural Resources, had called me down to her office on the Stanley waterfront. Statuesque, charismatic, with a sharp mind and a no-nonsense manner, I not only liked her but was slightly in awe of her.

'I know your contract is up, Joe, and Zoe will be filling your post.' Zoe Luxton was the Falklands' recently qualified home-grown vet. 'So I have a proposal for you. I'd like you to consider the position of Senior Veterinary Officer.'

I was touched, and in many ways it would be a dream come true. It would also mean a financially secure future. I had been enthralled by the island wildlife, the fishing vessels, long walks in fierce gales on pure sandy beaches, and the geniality of the Falklanders. But I was also saddened – because I was caught in the horns of a moral dilemma.

'Phyl, thank you so much. It means a lot. But I just don't think I can. My father's health is deteriorating, and my older brother Nick has been bearing the responsibility. I have to go back to the UK and support him.' I was vacillating. Sometimes it's harder to say 'no' in all its unforgiving finality.

'OK. Understood. Well, have a think about it and for now we'll leave it on the table. Keep me apprised of your decision.'

On the way home, I decided to fulfil a long-held ambition by flying to Punta Arenas in Patagonia and spending a couple of weeks travelling up the long, sinewy nation of Chile. Over the last five days I had explored the Atacama Desert, marvelled at the intense hues of the Altiplano, endured altitude sickness, revelled in the adobe *pueblos* with their touchingly simple limewashed churches, visited the saltpetre workings that had once made Iquique so fabulously wealthy, and just dropped off my hire truck in the fading evening light. Tomorrow, I would fly back down to Santiago then out to Rapa Nui – Easter Island – home of the mighty mo'ai.

I nipped into an internet café to check my messages, and there was an ominous email from my brother. 'Father's taken a turn for the worse and has been admitted to Derriford Hospital in Plymouth. Just driving down from Derby. Will take me four hours.' The email was only one hour old.

I had a gut feeling. I quickly googled the hospital phone number and booked an international call with the cashier. Outside, the traffic rumbled around the beautiful Plaza Arturo Prat, flanked by its extravagant medley of Moorish, Gothic and neoclassical architecture, all raised at great expense on the fortunes and egos of the nitrate barons. The call was put through, and the conversation quickly hit a rock.

'I'm so very sorry,' the nurse went on. 'Yes, he passed away peacefully half an hour ago. Is there anything I can do for you?'

I was the first to know. 'Just... please tell my brother I've been informed and I'm coming home straightaway. And thank you for being with my father.'

Damn him. Damn him for up and dying like that. I had selfishly taken a long overdue holiday on the rash assumption that he was doing all right, and allowed him to die alone. This was a guilt I would carry. I crossed the square, passing the elaborate clock tower, and sat down in the Restaurante La Protectora. Blurry eyed, I hung my head in shame over my coffee cup.

I was back in England within three days, and over the following weeks the offer of the top job in the Falklands slipped out of view, displaced by weightier matters. But it wasn't long before I was ready to escape the oppressive deluge of UK private practice and go back to the diversity of island vetting. So I wrote a speculative email.

I had heard of the strange, fascinating and largely unknown island of St Helena, where you arrived by swinging ashore on a

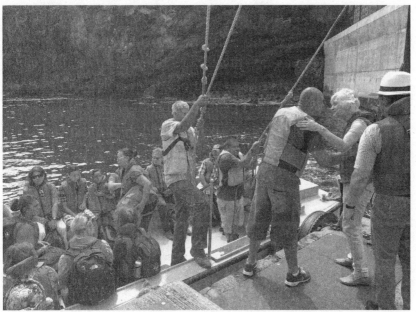

Landing and entering St Helena by rope at The Steps

rope. I had also met several Saint Helenians – 'Saints' – in the Falklands, and found them to be friendly, easy-going people.

St Helena is a volcanic remnant of the mid-Atlantic ridge lying some 1,300 miles from the nearest continent, Africa, and 2,000 miles from South America. Nothing in between. Beneath the water she is a Kilimanjaro, going down 5,000 metres or thereabouts into the abyssal depths of the Atlantic, but above the surface on the miserly forty-seven square miles of eroded summit, around 4,500 souls eke out an existence. I wanted to know more. Anyway, the island had me at 'swinging ashore on a rope'.

As emails go, it was a hard sell and I had little hope of its bearing fruit. I wrote to Andrew Gurr, Governor of St Helena, Ascension and Tristan da Cunha, a triad of UK Overseas Territories, offering my services like a street hawker, flogging my biosecurity, fisheries and general veterinary experience from the Falklands, where he too had served – as CEO. My appeal hinged on a momentous decision taken by the Whitehall mandarins in London: to retire the RMS *St Helena* and build an airport.

A BELOVED LIFELINE

For a long time, St Helena, the second remotest inhabited island in the world after its not-very-near neighbour Tristan da Cunha, had depended upon the lifeline of the RMS *St Helena* – known simply as 'the RMS', or affectionately by Captain Adam as 'Betty Blue Bucket' – the last true Royal Mail Ship.

The RMS didn't only carry mail, though she flew the mandatory red and white Post Office pennant from her masthead. She carried humanity and all its encumbrances: the sick and the terminally ill; the newlyweds and the newborn; the returning and departing friends and relatives separated or to be separated for years on end by the island's ongoing diaspora; the Technical Cooperation Officers that formed the hub of the expat community and provided the necessary professional expertise where there was a void; clergy of all creeds and diplomats of all competencies; judges and prisoners, even ex-cons who had served their time, perhaps eyeing the very same judge who had put them away over their morning bacon and eggs; haughty British government representatives and their puppyish junior acolytes; tourists both accidental and incidental lured by curiosity, a novel route home or a final entry on their bucket list; businessmen in pursuit of a lucrative deal, some benevolent and philanthropic, others with an eye to a quick buck; zealous conservationists enthralled by the endemicity of the island's flora and fauna; and PhD students hoping to crack open an unprecedented piece of research and forge a reputation. And cadavers: islanders who wished to add their mortal remains to the rich volcanic soils that reared them. To come home.

Then there was every conceivable item that modern living requires, from potatoes and nappies to chainsaws and bath plugs, along with a fair number of luxury items that aren't strictly necessary but certainly make life worthwhile, such as frozen croissants and maple syrup. And on occasion, sheep and chickens, which would one day be my own contribution to this eccentric and fascinating floating treasure house. If a ship could have a heart and soul, it would be her. Perhaps all those tragedies and joyful occasions that had played out on her many voyages had somehow left a vital residue in her iron body. Through all these associations – and there is no other way of saying it – the RMS *St Helena* was much loved.

Now, however, the island was planning to join the rest of the world by removing its reliance on the RMS and building an airport, with a barrowload of implications for biosecurity. The RMS yo-yoed between Cape Town 2,000 miles to the south-east of St Helena, and the UK military base of Ascension Island 800 miles to the north, voyages of days in either direction, and therefore she acted simultaneously as an incubator and a quarantine station. A disease carried on board could generally be relied upon to give itself away by cutting a swathe through the passengers, whether it be the common cold, chickenpox or a nasty bout of Ebola. In any event, there was a discreet contingency plan to anchor the ship out in St Helena's James Bay as a hospital in order to protect the island population while a pathogen ran its course. With the West African outbreak in 2014 there really was a threat of Ebola creeping in through this back door.

A plane is an altogether different proposition, with both the advantage and the danger of immediacy. It connects into international hubs, mingling people of all nations capable of harbouring all manner of diseases, and encapsulates a small piece of local atmosphere in the cabin and cargo holds that is vented as soon as the doors are opened on landing, with the potential to propel, for example, the tiger mosquito *Aedes albopictus*, vector of Zika, chikungunya, dengue and yellow fever, wholly intact and egg-laden, into the embracing warmth and humidity of St Helena's tropical maritime climate. Hence the veiled threat buried in my proposition – though it is not generally in my nature to threaten governors, which I suspect is probably somewhere on an antiquated statute as an overlooked hanging offence.

The Governor replied very courteously, promising to keep my email on file. Usually, that means consignment to the wastebin, physical or digital. But honourable Andrew Gurr was true to his word, and before long the Chief of Agriculture, Darren Duncan, phoned to recruit me on a six-month contract to train up some local paravets, since the island had no permanent veterinary surgeon.

So here I was, about to board the RMS bound for St Helena. My initial view of her was from the quayside of Georgetown, Ascension Island, the UK's all-seeing all-hearing military base shared with Cousin America. I was still bleary eyed after an overnight flight from RAF Brize Norton in Oxfordshire.

The ship was dinky but shapely, riding at anchor offshore in Clarence Bay. She had a cobalt blue hull, her chocolate anti-fouling showing just above the waterline, snow-white topsides, and a funnel the colour of Dijon mustard. For'ard on the cargo deck, a derrick was frantically stacking multicoloured containers like Lego; to the rear was the passenger area, peppered with portholes. Motorised pontoons and lighters buzzed back and forth, carrying stevedores, port officials and final provisions. Proudly maintained and somehow motherly, she was like a wise old hen drawing her many chicks in under her wings, providing warmth and safety from the hostility of the elements.

All aboard, with cargo nets, gangways and fenders securely stowed, the chain winch thunked and clattered throughout the hull as it broke out the anchor and the RMS gave three long blasts on the horn. She rounded the coarse and ragged lava flows on the north and east side of the island before leaving it behind bathed in the embers of an equatorial sunset. I watched the sun slipping behind Green Mountain on the aft deck and noticed a couple leaning against the taffrail. All the other passengers had wearied of the scene and gone to their cabins or the first sitting for dinner.

'Lovely evening,' I ventured. 'Why is it that people don't stay for the best bit?'

The man turned towards me, slim, dapper, with a snugly tailored suit, straight grey hair parted precisely to one side and a meticulously trimmed white moustache. It came as no surprise to learn later that he was a lover of classical music and a devout Baptist. 'Absolutely. It baffles me.' He extended a hand. 'Andrew Gurr.' He half turned. 'And Jean, my wife.'

'Governor Gurr?'

'That's the one. And you are?'

'Joe Hollins. I'm the vet. Actually, I have you to thank for being here.'

'Oh yes indeed, you wrote me that email. Glad to have you aboard. And I want to speak to you sometime about the care of the tortoises at Plantation House and the crayfish factory down on Tristan.' The tannoy crackled into life and a glockenspiel struck up with what would become a familiar call to feed, which I and all other passengers soon learned to respond to like Pavlov's dogs. The RMS was famous for its food, both quality and quantity, plied all day every day until belts demanded renotching. 'Ah – second sitting. We'll talk tomorrow.'

This serendipitous meeting gave me a front-row seat to the drama to come.

The RMS was delightfully old-fashioned, steeped in the traditions of the great P&O liners, her relaxed ambience partly owing to the fact that the two alternating crews and captains running the ship were nearly all Saints. It was their ship, and they were family and friends, with family and friends as passengers. Nothing could lend itself to a more convivial and caring atmosphere.

The dining room, warmly lit, portholed and expensively furnished with pristine white tablecloths and plush carpets, was the main scene of action. We were seated according to a table plan, with each assigned to an officer briefed to buy plentiful wine on the first night and stimulate the flow of inclusive conversation. In the centre was the captain's table, reserved for the captain and the notables – which included the Governor and his wife, of course – and waited on by a tall, handsome Saint in a cream waistcoat with brass buttons so polished they still flashed in the subdued lighting. This was Anthony 'Milktin' Thomas, a man whom I came to know well as a superb farmer with impeccable ethics and an impish sense of humour; every crew member had more than one role in life. Milktin was also my introduction to the amusing diversity of affectionate – often incident-linked – Saint nicknames, such as Ration Book, Purse Bag, Cold Slab, Small Change, Bread Belly, Fart Egg, Colonel Paint (talked a lot) and Bite The Dog (he did, after it bit him).

The dining room hummed with jollity, fuelled by drink and a seamless relay of mouth-watering dishes. Three days to St Helena, lavished with food, waited on hand and foot, and without a care in the world. What could be more escapist, more soothing for the soul? No one could have guessed that 800 miles away, someone was about to open a heavy and obstinate old door and, like an overeager potholer stumbling across a hibernating bear, disturb a lurking menace: a time capsule of latent death.

HARD ABOUT

The next day, our first full day at sea, I spent the morning chatting to the Governor on the aft deck. He was to be my first of five governors. Andrew Gurr was not a reared diplomat and unusually had been drawn into the service from the business sector. It was the Foreign Office's rationale that running a small island was not dissimilar to running a company and that his managerial acumen could prove very useful.

Towards lunchtime, an officer weaved his way towards us through the tables and umbrellas, his tropical whites glowing in the sear of the sun. He leaned down and whispered discreetly in the Governor's ear. 'Excuse me,' said the Governor, pushing back his plastic chair. 'Duty calls.'

He returned a different man, distracted and wearing a frown. Jean joined us and threw him an affectionate glance. 'So, you're really looking forward to getting back and sorting this one out?' she asked sarcastically.

'It's not quite that simple,' he replied glumly.

'Well,' I joked, 'she's your ship, I suppose. You could always turn her around.'

His reply flummoxed me. He hesitated, then stared vacantly into the sky. 'Yes... yes... I could do that. And that may be the solution.' I hadn't made a novel suggestion; it was clearly in the forefront of his mind. Or was he just being enigmatic? I dismissed my thoughts as fanciful. It was none of my business anyway. With that, the Governor stalked off and for the rest of the day, he was nowhere to be seen.

After dinner, a few of us settled into the hypnotically beautiful evening, sipping Drambuie on the aft deck, the laid teak under our feet vibrating to the thrust of the twin propellors. We watched the white wake trailing into the blackness, beneath a crescent moon with a million stars in a flawless firmament. It is hard to beat the soothing caress of a balmy tropical night at sea.

Our soporific mood was rudely shattered by a long blast on the ship's horn. It was entirely incongruous, like a belligerent drunk at a ballet. But it had the desired effect. It jolted everybody into utter silence. Seven of those and we'd be sinking and manning the lifeboats, but no other blast followed to pierce the emptiness. Still, something was wrong. I sat up ramrod straight.

The tannoy crackled into life. It was Captain Rodney Young, also known, in the witty Saint tradition, as Schoolbus.

'This is the captain speaking,' he began, his voice ponderous and full of foreboding. 'I have an important announcement to make.' He paused for effect. The passengers were as motionless as mannequins. 'Today, on St Helena, a large hundred-year-old bomb was found along with boxes marked "EXPLOSIVE" in a tower above Jamestown.' Gasps and exclamations. 'After discussion with the authorities we have been advised that there is a suitably qualified bomb disposal expert on Ascension Island. It has therefore been decided that the only option is to turn the ship around and return to collect this person so that the bomb can be made safe. We will make full steam using both engines and estimate that we will reach Ascension by late tomorrow afternoon. We will not drop anchor but immediately turn the ship back on a heading for St Helena. I apologise for the delay that this will entail.' Again, a pause. 'The ship,' he then continued with a distinct flair for the dramatic, 'will commence turning.'

And turn it did, at full speed. The deck cambered, the moon and stars wheeled swiftly and surreally to starboard, and the propellors thrashed out a billowing arc of wake that in no time looped back on itself. A crescendo of excited chatter broke out.

I later learned that archaeologist Ben Jeffs had been contracted to do a stocktake of the island's built heritage which, thanks to the paranoia and deep coffers of the East India Company, is extensive. Overhanging the brim of the V-shaped ravine that cradles Jamestown, beyond Ladder Hill Fort and the gun emplacements, stands a lone Martello tower with a large bronze door at its base. Jeffs had wrestled with the door, keen to examine the internal condition of the tower and see if it held any treasures fit for the island museum. With a bit of judiciously applied force, it had finally given way but, as his eyes adjusted to the dim light within, his eager anticipation had evaporated. The treasures he saw filled him with horror.

'It's not just one bomb,' the Governor confided, 'rather it appears to be a large cache of munitions. And it's pretty much exactly where we had a recent serious rockfall.'

Rockfall: the inherited fear of every Jamestown resident, an ever-present threat of death poised above their heads. Jamestown is so tightly squeezed into its long, tapering ravine that it looks for all the world as if the streets have been poured into a mould, the colourful little stone cottages lapping up the sides of the precipitous slopes. These slopes are steep, shattered lava flows with a sparse sprinkling of scrub, torn through by eight million years of dogged erosion; water is constantly nibbling away at the cracks and crevices, further breaking up and destabilising the rock. Just six months earlier, a 300-tonne rockfall swept through the Baptist chapel, demolishing half of the building and killing a dog, and bouncing boulders the size of pumpkins across the

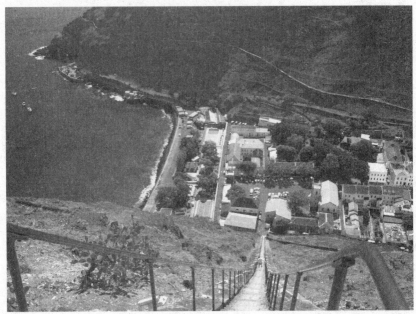

Jamestown seen from the top of Jacob's Ladder

road into the children's playground. In 1984, a mother and child were killed in their cottage at the head of the valley. And famously – in Jamestown at least – on 17 April 1890, 1,500 tonnes of rock destroyed fourteen houses, killing nine people.

Several months after my arrival, I made a house visit to treat a sick cat belonging to an archetypal sweet old lady living in a tiny, linear cottage wedged between the other historic structures of lower Jamestown. Her access was down a narrow alley, where her front door, set into a high stone wall, gave on to a central passageway with rooms coming off it on either side. In the passageway, blocking two thirds of it, sat a pram-sized boulder. I asked her what it was doing there.

'Ah that! It came through the roof of my living room one year. Luckily, I was in bed with the cat.' She seemed stoically indifferent to the perennial threat of annihilation from above. I asked her why it was still there, and she let out a delightful cackle. 'Oh now, my lovely, look around. We'd have to knock down half of Jamestown to get it out. And I like it. Sometimes I sit on it and have a cup of tea.' Just revenge on the boulder, I thought, hugely amused.

Since then, the UK government, to its great credit, has spent millions securing the sides of the ravine with avalanche netting, employing the very best for such a task: the French. The flanks are now silvered in sheets of galvanised mesh, lashed together over the contours like a hairnet. The rockfalls have been caged and tamed.

But that is now. Then, the apparent munitions stash in the Martello tower above the densest part of historic Jamestown appeared to be a very real threat and had to be taken seriously. Not least because decaying munitions can be bad tempered; like old men, they don't like to be moved and tend to explode.

Just before dusk we pulled into Clarence Bay, where Ascension's Administrator was waiting on a launch to meet us. But of the promised bomb disposal expert, there was no sign. The gangway was lowered and the Governor whisked away to the town. Clearly there was some hierarchical jousting going on.

Expectantly, the passengers lined the railings, but as the hours ticked by, speculation broke out. A rumble told us that Captain Rodney had dropped anchor, a bad omen. Meanwhile, a pod of pantropical dolphins amazed and entertained us with their cunning method of driving flying fish towards the brightly lit hull, where the ethereally winged but foolhardy fish, zipping through the night air at tremendous speed, stunned themselves with fatal 'thoks' against the steel wall and served themselves up as dolphin dinners.

Our dinners, first and second sitting, also came and went. A bunch of diehards, including myself, hung out late on the aft deck until, just before midnight, the putter of a launch could be heard across the water. It delivered the Governor, Flight Lieutenant Caroline Crowson – the bomb disposal expert, and the wife of the Base Commander, who seemed to be out for a jolly to St Helena. We broke into applause, and the Governor glanced up with an appreciative nod. The anchor was whipped out of the seabed, the RMS put about, and both engines engaged at full speed for St Helena.

The next day I bumped into the Governor at my favourite airy hangout, the starboard wing of the bridge, the bow wave surging past way beneath us.

'The bastards!' he muttered, trying to maintain his usual restraint. 'They wouldn't give her to me. Me – the Governor!' I could hear the lingering incredulity in his voice. 'I tried to contact Whitehall but on a Saturday night, of course, nobody was there. Then the Commander of the British Forces of the South Atlantic Islands in the Falklands got involved. We wrangled and tossed and turned the matter over but they wouldn't budge.'

The Governor's eyes sparkled with triumph and his moustache bristled. 'Then I had a brainwave.'

The conversation had gone something like this:

'Just a minute', said the Governor, struck by a thought. 'Am I not the Queen's representative? Don't I hold the rank of Commander-in-Chief?'

'Er – yes,' replied the Commander of the British Forces of the South Atlantic Islands, somewhat reluctantly.

'So... doesn't that mean I outrank you?'

The subordinate commander had been rumbled, and with an audible sigh he replied: 'Yes, it does.'

'Well, why on earth didn't you tell me?'

'You didn't ask, sir.'

'I didn't ask?' (I imagine here an expletive, but as a god-respecting man and a diplomat, the Governor may have bitten his tongue.) 'Right, then! What must I do to get you to agree?'

'Sir, you have to task me.'

'Task you? Very well then. I task you to hand over your bomb disposal expert.'

The order of command is sacrosanct in the armed services. 'Very well, sir.'

It was as simple as that. I roared with laughter. Bastards indeed. But sticklers for hierarchy.

Flight Lieutenant Crowson had a wretched time. She was confined to her cabin with seasickness the whole voyage. I wondered if this was the true reason for the initial refusal to travel, and perhaps explains why she never joined the Royal Navy.

THE ISLAND OF ST HELENA

St Helena at last.

The ship, delayed by the diplomatic duel, pulled into the anchorage during the early hours of Tuesday morning, dropped anchor and gave a single long blast on the horn to let the island know she was home. It was a sound that reverberated through the valleys and lifted islanders' hearts, the halloo of a mother's homecoming.

Passengers lined the handrails and pointed to the skyline, to the solitary Martello tower clinging to the lip of the ravine. There was the culprit. A rockfall from there would be merciless.

The maritime gateway to St Helena is as impressive as it is intentionally daunting. Coarse, angry cliffs rise like wings on either side of Jamestown, a mostly intact Georgian town of pretty stone buildings. From the waterfront, the sole entry to the island is via a single archway punched through a thick curtain wall of massive proportions which runs from flank to flank of the ravine, embracing the Castle with its fluttering Union Jack. Serried ranks of further, precisely constructed defensive walls, gun emplacements, forts and towers bristle on both sides, while the imperious citadel of High Knoll Fort threatens to crush the enemy from above.

St Helena was formerly the prized possession of the East India Company, a mighty trading institution whose ships and personnel outnumbered those of the Crown. She had been their base and their strategic hold on the world. The EIC poured its wealth into making the island, already a natural fortress with her colossal, sea-girt cliffs and steep, narrow valleys, into the most heavily fortified place on the planet. Every valley mouth was sealed off with a wall, every approach overlooked by a battery of cannon, and the prominences of her forty-seven square miles were interconnected with lookouts, semaphores and signal guns. One thing they couldn't build, though, was a dock, because of the steep, unstable seabed and the phenomenon of massive devastating rollers generated annually by northern pressure systems.

A lighter, *The Gannet*, ferried us to the Steps, tucked beneath the northern cliffs and the brooding, crab-like structure of a Victorian gun emplacement. And I was not to be disappointed; from a galvanised frame hung a row of thick, grippy ropes for swinging ashore, and a surge was on so that the boat bucked and chivvied like a restless colt in a stable. An assistant ashore swung a rope to the first waiting passenger, telling them when to take the leap, their outstretched hands making sure that there was no 'slip twixt cup and lip', which in real terms meant not being ground into fish food between the boat's leaping hull and the barnacled quayside.

Buried into the cliff face to dodge the falling rocks, a ribbon of brightly painted, historic stone buildings, strung out along the thin waterfront, led me to a road bridge crossing a wide dry moat to the Arch. Two vast wooden doors pinned back against high iron railings were crowned by the arms and motto of the East India Company, *Under the auspices of the King and the Senate of England*. The oversizing of everything reeked of historic might.

Beyond the arch lay a large, rectangular open space: the Grand Parade, where the EIC and afterwards, the Crown, mustered and drilled their troops. Flanking the Parade were the Castle; the inevitable mounted cannon; the law courts; the museum; the cavernous merchant warehouses; St James, the oldest Anglican church in the southern hemisphere, joined, as if in absolution, to the quaint, balconied cottage-front of Her Majesty's Prison; the 699 thigh-bruising steps of Jacob's Ladder in a vertiginous straight run 600 feet up to a flagged, cross-jacked ship's mast by a fort; and the shady Castle Gardens, with monuments and fountains, lilac-flowering jacarandas and aged banyan trees. The upper side of Grand Parade gave on to the broad Main Street, straight as a die and lined by pastel-coloured Georgian buildings with stone steps and iron-pillared balconies, as intact, they say, as when Wellington – and the captive Napoleon – stepped ashore: the one, no doubt, jauntily, the other with lead in his boots (not wellingtons...). It was all a little shabby, but nevertheless magnificent. A film set begging for a crew.

'You're impressed then?' Darren Duncan, tall and willowy, long faced and square jawed, was the Chief of Agriculture and Natural Resources, otherwise known as the CANRO – my new boss. A lapsed Seventh Day Adventist, he was polite and soft spoken, insightful and supportive, with a repository of knowledge that calmly cut through any nonsense and an unbreakable honesty that could be relied upon. I soon came to realise how lucky I was to be under his command, and he became a staunch friend.

'I'm completely blown away. It's a gem. Really beautiful.'

'Yes, we got a little left behind out here, but we like it. OK, the plan for today. First a yellowfin tuna roll at Anne's – freshly caught of course – then...' he tossed me a set of car keys, 'you're going to have your first experience of Ladder Hill Road.' This, I was to discover, was the tight, often single-track stonewalled road that snakes up, or rather hangs off, the side of the ravine, offering a route to the interior of the island. 'Work can wait until tomorrow.'

Flight Lieutenant Crowson, meanwhile, was on the clock and put straight to her task. Doubtless togged up in her protective body armour, she let herself in to the base of the Martello tower to find that the wooden boxes stencilled 'EXPLOSIVE' were these days mere stage props: empty. But the bomb was real enough: a rusty, spherical cartoon bomb the size of a medicine ball that should have had a fizzing fuse hanging from its stopper and 'ACME BOMBS' stencilled around its waist; only this was an airburst bomb dating from the Boer War and entirely serious in its purpose.

She wisely told the authorities that the bomb greatly preceded any training she had received and needed specialist attention, then she cased it in a metal box, and assured Jamestonians that should it explode, the strongly built Martello tower would contain it – although the common belief was that it would more probably quarry out the clifftop. Negotiations began with the Foreign Office for an expert in Victorian munitions, a sort of UXB antiquarian, to come and neutralise the threat.

INTO THE INTERIOR

The offices of Agriculture and Natural Resources at Scotland, formerly and less confusingly Scott's Land and not at all Celtic, is the only outlying part of the St Helena Government, set quite appropriately for its role near the middle of the island. Encountering the island's interior on that first visit, I properly understood the description of St Helena that I'd heard so many times: 'an emerald set in bronze'.

The outer two-thirds of the island is, for the most part, a tortured and arid, caramel-coloured volcanic land stripped of native bush and topsoil by centuries of foraging goats and men wielding axes, the one as irresponsible as the other. Even in the 1700s they knew they had a problem. It was said that, at times, heavy rainfall turned the sea to chocolate as eight million years' worth of rich organic matter was consigned to the seabed, never to be reclaimed. Officially, this coastal perimeter is called the Crown Wastes, but despite the derogatory name it is a landscape of spectacular naked geology.

The interior stands in such huge contrast to the perimeter that it takes every newcomer by surprise: rich, verdant fields crowned by peaks of endemic cloud forest, with swathes of commercial woodland embossing the ridges and upper valleys. The winding, grass-banked, single-track lanes, reminiscent of the byways of Devon, with their pedantic, lichen-stained finger posts displaying fractions of a mile, leave the traveller in no doubt of a resolutely British influence.

St Helena is a tropical island with a sub-tropical, maritime climate, which is warm, moist and frost free: an incubator climate, perfect for animals, fruit and vegetables and every pest and disease that bedevils them. It is a sort of brittle Eden. Scotland, which as it turned out would be my place of work for years to come, is a well-tended former plantation, with offices surrounded by flower beds and banana trees, and cultivated terraces running down to Conservation, where ingenious Kew-trained horticulturalists pull endemic species back from the brink of extinction and fight the relentless march of the greedy invasives. It is, altogether, a delightful working environment.

My team of trainee paravets were Arthur, Roberta, Patrice, Clayton 'Chopsie', Rico 'Turby' and Cardinal; good and willing students all. Course notes and written tests are important, but the best training always comes from hard-won, hands-on experience. Yet cases can't be ordered up like dishes on a Chinese menu; they're random. As it happened, though, over my six-month contract the calls came in thick and fast. Some were more than ordinary, and they mainly, but not exclusively, involved cattle.

THE MALEVOLENT RAYS

'Cooper's got a cow with a bad eye down at Luffkins, Joe.'

A bad eye indeed, and a textbook classic: squamous cell carcinoma, an aggressive and malignant cancer caused by ultraviolet light in cattle with unpigmented eyelids. And cats, come to that. And an unfortunate pink-eared sheep I happened to see that I rapidly made earless. St Helena is blasted by UV light, even when overcast. The eye was cruelly distorted by the aggressive tumour, and the cow was clearly in a hideous amount of pain. She'd lost considerable weight, with the added complication that she had a young, dependent calf at foot.

'Cooper.' I addressed the old Saint farmer who stood beside me in his faded blue overalls. 'The only thing to try is to remove her eye, but there's a risk. She's down in condition.'

'That's OK,' he replied, his trust and acceptance refreshing. 'She'll lose her calf anyway if we do nothing.'

It was a full team effort. I had to have her deeply sedated, and in cattle there's a real danger of regurgitation, as bringing up the cud is part and parcel of being a ruminant. In a small, corrugated iron shed with an earthen floor, we wove a casting hitch around her body and legs, then I knocked her down with an intravenous bolus of the versatile sedative xylazine.

'Chopsie, pillow under her head, please. Keep that neck up in case she regurgitates. Protect the good eye underneath, it can chafe. Patrice, lay out the kit. Roberta, scrub up as an assistant, the bucket and povidone antiseptic is over there. Arthur, inject her with the antibiotic and painkiller, please. Cardie, sit on her rump in case she wakes up and tries to stand.'

I pumped the back of the eyeball with local, stitched the eyelids together and made an elliptical cut around the whole. It was a slow and tricky dissection, the kit a mixed bag of ancient surgical instruments, the scissors frustratingly blunt and mangling my fingers, the tissue tough and defiant. Sweat ran down my forehead. But I was committed. The whole eyeball along with lids and all its secretory glands had to be removed, as well as the offending malignancy. At last, the eyeball came free, a grotesque and gory tennis ball. I closed everything up and stitched a pad over the site to control post-op swelling.

Back aching, I sat back on my haunches with a huge sigh of relief. My students were revelling in it all, a good sign. 'And now I'll show you some magic,' I said mysteriously, waving a prepared syringe in the air. Normally, we let a bovine sedative slowly wear off, though there is always the danger of a broken leg or a dislo-cated hip when 400 kilos of hallucinating cow does a drunken waltz. But I had been clearing out drugs from the enormous storeroom and come across some overstocked antidote for a related sedative, usually used in small quantities for dogs and cats. 'This,' I announced a little dramatically, 'is probably fifty pounds' worth, but we don't care because we've got far too much of it. Prepare to be amazed.' I injected the antidote into her rump, and within minutes she was standing and looking for her calf, a far safer recovery all round. My students gazed on in amazement. The magic of modern medicine. Five hundred years ago, I would have been burned at the stake for less.

Within weeks, the cow regained her weight, the relief from pain made evident, and the calf, a heifer, grew up to one day replace her.

AN OILY ARSE

'Message at Reception, Joe. Gary's steer has drunk a tub of old sump oil over at Farm Buildings.'

'What?' This was a first. Farm Buildings was a mixed site of abattoir, piggery, livestock pens and car-repair workshop. It sounded as if the last two had become confused.

This was my first meeting with Gary 'Bullfrog' Stevens, a Buddha of a man with a singsong voice and a generosity of spirit like no other. I would later learn that he had an endearing habit of pulling a bottle of rum out from behind his passenger seat, along with a couple of cups. An industrious farmer with many irons in the fire, his love for the island resonated in his every word, the very soil surely flowing in his veins for blood. It turned out the steer hadn't just drunk the tarry black sump oil, it had savoured every last drop and licked the tub dry.

'Why on earth, Gary, would it do such a crazy thing?'

'I don't know, lurvie. I suppose it must have tasted good,' he chortled. 'I prefer a rum and Coke.' His warmth and sense of humour were contagious.

'For all I know, there could be brake fluid, thinners, all sorts in there.' The tame steer watched us calmly with its innocent round eyes, completely indifferent to our concern and proffering an oily black muzzle in evidence. 'Well, it doesn't seem much bothered.'

Nonetheless, I made up a generous mixture of activated charcoal, stomach-tubed the steer, and proceeded to splatter every participant with black sludge as I battled with the overflowing funnel, the flailing tube, and a perfectly well but now thoroughly indignant animal.

At the end of it all, Gary stood back and roared with laughter. 'Lurvie,' he said, between snorts, 'we all look like coalminers.'

A few days later, I caught up with Gary and asked him how the calf was doing.

'The calf?' he repeated in an amused, high-pitched voice. 'Never looked back. Only thing is, it's been shitting black ever since and I've never seen such an oily arse.' And he laughed and I laughed and we both laughed together.

MARCH OF THE CATERPILLARS

'Joe, Solomons have got a sick bullock down at Broad Bottom.'

Broad Bottom was a tumbling swathe of pasture and an old flax mill owned by the largest company on the island, Solomons of Jamestown.

The bullock was puzzling; it appeared to be blind, had lost its senses, and was drooling thick, glutinous ropes of saliva from its muzzle. A hasty and potentially finger-crushing examination of the oral cavity achieved nothing more than coating me in gloop, as if I had been assaulted by a giant land snail. Cattle produce mind-boggling quantities of saliva, over 100 litres a day, lubricating the cud and nourishing the rumen. Finally, the penny dropped: this animal couldn't swallow; its throat was paralysed. Along with the incoordination, the loss of vision and the mental derangement – and dismissing the alarming possibility of bovine spongiform encephalopathy, more commonly known as mad cow disease, because it had no right to be on this speck of an island – I came to the one remaining conclusion.

'It's poisoned!' But what on earth with?

'Armyworm,' murmured Arthur at my elbow. 'It must be army-worm.' Arthur, craggy-faced and close to retirement, had a lifetime's agricultural experience. In his spare time, he preached at the Apostolic Church, and was gifted with an ability to conjure up arcane and witty sayings, usually delivered with a hefty dose of sarcasm.

'What in god's name is an armyworm?'

'Not really a worm. More a moth.' He pointed at an extensive patch of distant pasture that was the colour of hay and perfectly delineated from the abundant green sward all around. 'See that

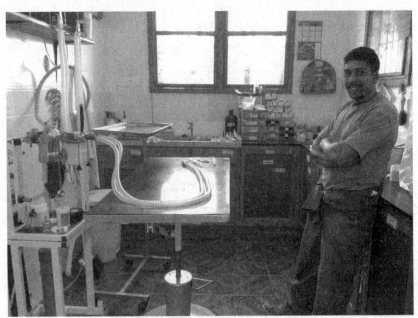

Veterinary assistant Rico Williams at our clinic

grass yonder, all dead and yellowed? Like someone spilled their gruel? That's armyworm.'

'It's an army of moths then?'

'Well... not really a moth. More the moth's babies. They cut the shoots and kill the grass. And sometimes the cattle.'

'You mean caterpillars? The caterpillars kill the cattle?' I asked incredulously. Was this folklore or something real? 'How?'

'I thought you might tell me,' he replied drily, and with some justification.

I had never heard of this and yet I took him at his word; there is no substitute for local knowledge accrued over generations. The animal was hopelessly lost, but at least I could try to answer the mystery of the cattle-murdering caterpillars. It was true that in recent days, walking through certain areas of thigh-high grass, I had noticed the clouds of dully coloured moths that rose around me like windblown confetti. I sought out a good patch of armyworm and parted the dead strands of grass. The open roots were writhing with small green caterpillars, waxy brown pupae scattered among them.

A deep trawl on the internet finally came up with the answer. *Spodoptera* moths are ravishers of grassland – at least, their 'babies' are – with sometimes terrible consequences for rural African communities. It was only recently understood why armyworm occasionally kills cattle. Certain grasses have a defence mechanism against attack: cyanogenesis. They make cyanide. And top of the list was the African grass much favoured for pasture on St Helena, kikuyu. It turns out that the caterpillars, and the cattle too, have a degree of resistance to cyanide, and peripatetic grazing never causes the cattle to ingest enough cyanide to harm them. The dead grass, though, was an altogether different matter: the cyanide became concentrated in lethal doses. It was a rural Agatha Christie plot with bovine victims.

I filled the team in on the fascinating details and complimented Arthur on his knowledge. His face took on a wry, faintly amused expression: 'Well... I wasn't pissed up against the wall and hatched by the sun, you know!'

There was no answer to that.

NO FLUFFY BUNNIES

My time on St Helena was drawing to a close. Six months had passed, and my students had excelled. We'd had a decent spectrum of clinical cases, neutered dogs and cats, trimmed donkeys' hooves, fought Weil's disease, inseminated goats, stomach-pumped rat-poisoned dogs, sutured abscessed cats, fixed fractured limbs, taken revelatory X-rays, peered down microscopes at parasites, incubated chicken and turtle eggs, hoisted recumbent cows in slings, and learned about the myriad wonders of the mammalian body and its failings. And I hadn't restricted myself to the brief but addressed all veterinary issues on the island and drawn up an exhaustingly long report. 'The only thing is,' I pronounced carelessly one day, 'we haven't had a decent calving.' Arthur cupped both hands over the knotty end of his favourite stick and, like a Congolese shaman, murmured something dark, eyed me ruefully and slowly shook his head. I had summoned up a demon.

It was sluicing down with rain and had been for days when the call came in. 'Rodney "Eggshell" up at Pouncey's says his neighbour has a cow with a stuck calf. And he says she's wild.'

Pouncey's is high up and receives more than its fair share of rainfall. Eggshell met us at the bottom of his track, and we clambered, crawled and clawed our way across a bog, the mud sucking at our boots and the rain pounding off our backs.

Finally, in the field, we came upon a furious cow, the monstrous disfigurement of a swollen head protruding from her vulva. Eggshell's neighbour had lassoed her neck and tethered her between two thorn trees, but her hind quarters still swung from side to side like a hellish pendulum, intent on breaking my arm. No cattle crush to hold her, no bar to protect me from being kicked into another realm. But a reassuring rule of thumb is that usually a calving cow won't kick. I just hoped she had read the rule book.

'OK, everyone, this one's a classic,' I shouted through the mayhem of weather with my hand still exploring her vagina and the malpresentation. 'Dead calf, swollen head, both legs back, and the vagina bone dry. It won't go backwards, it won't go forwards and it's impossible to reach the legs. The only way to save the cow and retrieve the calf is to...'

'Cut off the head.'

'Yup, 'fraid so...' Her vengeful tail lashed my face, choking off my words and splattering me with blood and faeces. I spat out the salty concoction and blinked the debris from my stinging eyes. 'I guess I deserved that,' I croaked. Anyway, what did it matter? By now I was plastered in an ungodly mixture of rain, mud, blood, faeces and foetal fluids.

Carefully guarding a scalpel blade between my fingers to avoid slashing the vulva, I worked my way into the calf's neck, severing the muscles and tendons and finally separating the cervical vertebrae. The head came away and hit the mud at my feet with a grisly plop. I automatically kicked it to one side and pushed the body of the calf back into the resisting chamber of the womb, then sank in armpit deep to grapple for the legs. I battled with the faraway hooves, constantly slipping from my fingertips, my arm bloodless, bruised and aching. Several litres of hot, steaming liquid hosed my chest and ran down my body, filling my trousers and boots. I sighed. Of course, urine, the missing ingredient. Why not? Besides, it was warming on a cold day.

Eventually, I succeeded in cupping each hoof in the palm of my hand and straightening out the legs. The team fell to it with calving ropes and the invaluable calving jack, and the unfortunate decapitated calf was delivered, the cow saved.

'A bull calf,' I pronounced sadly, looking under the calf's belly. As ever, I felt mixed emotions at being unable to save a newborn animal, even in order to spare its mother. But where there's livestock there's deadstock, as they say in rural Yorkshire.

However, in a classic moment of hubris, the cow hadn't finished with us yet. There was an ominous, mucousy, slurping sound behind me as if a giant squid had fallen from a tree, followed by exclamations of shocked surprise from my students. I swung round. Oh no. Not that.

'Her bed's out,' said Eggshell, in a fatalistic monotone. Her whole womb, flaccid after hours of straining, had prolapsed out of her body, thirty kilos of quivering pink flesh that should never see the light of day. It was now also plastered in mud.

I sent Roberta across the bog for some more kit and braced myself for the next battle. I looked at my team, bedraggled but still keen, possibly even enjoying the unexpected turn of events.

'OK. Bonus lesson – unfortunately. The impossible art of squeezing a quart into a pint pot.' Cliché or not, it was no exaggeration: a prolapsed bovine uterus is inside out and has a ghastly propensity to double in size, like leavening dough.

But there is a trick. First, an epidural. I worked the tail like a pump handle and felt for the telltale divot, then slipped in the local anaesthetic. The tail went limp and she began to sway. 'Now we have to frogleg her.' An almighty wrestling match ensued with the back end of the cow, the front end doing its best to resist us, but eventually chemistry won over bovine obstinacy, and we got her down on her belly fully froglegged. It's a position that creates a sort of vaginal suction, a giant, anatomical vacuum cleaner.

I kneeled behind her and encircled the bloated, bloody doughball in my arms, cradling it in my lap then using my whole body like a cider press, fingers probing madly around the vulva to work in the slippery tissue. The task always feels hopeless but the key is patience. Gradually it shrank and began to slide, then suddenly and gratifyingly fell back in the way it had come. My arm in up to the armpit once more, I stretched out my fingers and reinverted the telescoped horns of the womb. Some vets use the neck of a wine bottle, by preference a slope-shouldered Beaujolais, and although I was more than ready to empty one, none were at hand. Finally, some sturdy stitches around the vulva stented with tubing ensured that we didn't have to return and do it all over again tomorrow. Worried that she'd chill in the mud and the rain, we then rolled, levered, dragged, and generally fought with the ungrateful beast until by some miracle we had her in the relative comfort of a garden shed.

I returned home sodden to the core, stinking like a midden, and multihued with excrement, mud and blood. I staggered into the wet room and stood under a hot, revitalising shower fully clothed. Teeny took one look at me, threw back her blonde hair in horror, and paled. 'Oh my god.

Where's the massacre?'

And some students think it's all fluffy bunnies.

TRUMPING THE DEVIL

The day before Teeny and I left, the RMS anchored in the bay and waiting to carry us both off, a Land Rover pulled up in the yard. The bulky figure of Gary Stevens clambered out, and between the fingers of his ham-sized hand – 'No bugger ever made a glove for these beauties,' he'd say – he brandished an old St Helenian £1 note. 'So that you don't forget us, lurvie.'

I heard him swallow his words and saw his reddened eyes. A big man with a big heart. I was deeply moved. I gripped him by the shoulder. 'Who knows, Gary? Maybe I'll be back one day. I hope so.'

A few months later, on a dark and bitter winter's night in the Wiltshire town of Hungerford, I stood on a snow-rimed station platform seeing Darren Duncan off on a train. He'd been holidaying in the UK with his girlfriend Freda, and we'd spent a couple of days at my cottage enjoying pub lunches and country walks crunching through the drifts. As the train screeched into the platform, we hugged our farewells, and he hefted his luggage.

'Oh, by the way,' he said, turning his head as he reached for the carriage door, his breath steaming in the icy air, 'we're going to advertise for the first permanent vet.' He climbed up into the carriage. 'I'd apply if I was you.' And with that short phrase, he reshaped my future.

And the bomb? What became of the bomb? The diplomatic tussle with the Foreign Office became typically mired in politics and talk of who should pick up the tab. But the Jamestown fire brigade showed good old-fashioned common sense. Several of them remembered playing around the bomb as children – making a mockery of my train set – and knew it well. Tiring of the drawn-out, expat diplomatic shenanigans, they came up with a pragmatic solution: they picked it up, drove it away and threw it into the sea.

Sometimes it's the simplest solution that trumps the Devil.

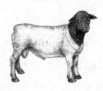

FOR WANT OF A TROUGH

A ship, an isle, a sickle moon –
With few but with how splendid stars
The mirrors of the sea are strewn
Between their silver bars!

James Elroy Flecker

THE OLD BLUNDERBUSS

Andrew Greentree, Royal Mail Ship captain number two, crouched down on one knee and placed the heavy, steel muzzle of the antique weapon against the furry forehead.

'Watch the recoil, Andrew. Both hands and bend your elbows slightly. It kicks like a bloody mule.' As I already knew to my cost. 'And a little higher above the eyes. Angle it down. Aim for the neck.'

He pulled back the cocking pin, cupped his right hand in his left, and squeezed the trigger, his face screwing up as he anticipated the discharge of the .22 calibre cartridge. There was a loud 'pock', a puff of gunpowder smoke, and he jerked backwards.

'Perfect.' I inserted a screwdriver into the neatly punched hole to show him the angle of his shot. 'Right into the frontal lobes. Sheep have a surprisingly small brain, it's easy to miss. And the worst thing to do is aim too low and ventilate their sinuses. And remember that it's only a stun gun. You still have to cut the throat to ensure death. Three more to go.'

'Lovely,' said Captain Andrew with characteristic dry humour. 'Schoolbus,' he continued, referring to Captain Rodney, 'has already teased me that I've come ashore to learn how to kill dead sheep.'

Before him lay a macabre coconut shy: four glassy-eyed sheep heads, evenly spaced, propped up in the deep grass at the back of the offices. I had collected them from the local abattoir and stored them in my freezer to await Andrew's arrival; defrosting them overnight on the kitchen floor had created a pool of blood worthy of a murder scene.

What he held in his hands was the oldest captive-bolt pistol I had ever seen, also called a humane stun gun. We had four of the latest Accles & Shelvoke 'CASH' pistols in the vet office, neat, cushioned devices for the humane slaughter of livestock, but this one, which belonged to the RMS *St Helena*, was an absolute beast.

The RMS was about to make one of her biannual trips to the UK, a sixteen-day voyage across 5,000 nautical miles of ocean. Among her many other functions she was also an ark, and throughout her career had carried animals in her livestock pen tucked under the foredeck over the chain lockers. I had a plan to take advantage of the voyage to shift the make-up of the island sheep flocks to a breed more appropriate for the muggy climate: a hair sheep called the Dorper. I would board the ship and, on arrival in Portland, Dorset, oversee the loading of some pedigree rams and ewes, along with sixty parent-stock chickens. Then I would take a few weeks' leave in the UK, having transformed the RMS into a floating farmyard.

Since I would be absent for the return leg, in the event of a tragedy, the captain had the burdensome responsibility of ending any animal suffering, and for this reason the RMS carried a captive-bolt pistol in the captain's cabin safe. Captain Rodney had the up voyage, and Captain Andrew the down voyage, so Andrew needed to know how to use it. In fact, he was legally required to. The ship had an Animal Transporter Certificate issued by the UK ministry and it plugged into a weighty chunk of EU legislation which demanded: 'a means of killing suitable for the species shall be available to the attendant or a person on board who has the necessary skill to perform this task humanely and efficiently'. It also meant potentially that he would have to wring the neck of an ailing chicken.

My plan was a good plan, a complex plan, and I had thrashed out the logistics of getting four livestock trailers carrying eleven quarantined sheep from eight widely scattered farmers to converge on the port early on departure day in almost paranoid, forensic detail. What could possibly go wrong?

When Captain Andrew had learned of his added responsibility, he contacted me from the ship. 'Joe, I think you need to see this thing and take it ashore to try it out. It looks positively ancient.'

I cleared island immigration, startling customs with the information that I was about to return with a pistol and live ammunition, and took the ferry out into the bay where the ship rode gently at anchor. The jovial uniformed officers, the bustle of the ship, and the smell of breakfast wafting up from the galley lifted my spirits. I always relished being aboard this lovely vessel. The Chief Officer, Peter Milton, took me up onto the bridge.

Captain Andrew was at his desk filling in paperwork. 'Welcome, Joe. Take a seat.' He reached down to a small safe tucked under a cabinet and drew out a weighty cloth bag. 'Here's the pistol.'

'Not for deranged passengers then?' I always wondered if it was true that a captain kept a handgun for mutiny, piracy and lunacy.

'No. That's the other one,' he joked. I think.

I pulled out the gun in something akin to awe. It was a museum piece with a sinister beauty: a fat mahogany pistol grip, darkened to ebony by gun oil and hand grease; a gleaming bronze body the colour of rancid butter; and a hefty gunmetal-blue muzzle that rotated to lock in the cartridge. Stamped deeply into the bronze were the words 'COX UNIVERSAL KILLER BROMLEY KENT'; the marrying of a weapon of destruction to the sedate, leafy suburbs of the Garden of England seemed incongruous, to say the least. It came with a faded cardboard packet of .22 calibre cartridges and a crumbling instruction leaflet. It must have been at least sixty years old.

OOPS

'Here.' Ken Henry, veterinary and livestock assistant, handed me a short plank of wood. 'See if it still works.'

The recommended technique to test a stun gun is to fire into a wooden plank, as to air fire provides no back resistance to the bolt and batters the gun's inner components. And 'captive bolt' means just that: there is no bullet to ricochet. But OK, yes, perhaps I shouldn't have tried it out in the office.

I placed the plank at my feet, pushed in a very out-of-date .22 cartridge and rotated the locking mechanism, then, clamping the oversized mahogany pistol grip in both hands, pulled the side-trigger.

The pistol discharged with a loud explosion. The windows rattled, the plank flew apart in opposite directions, fragments of concrete shot across the room like miniature ballistic missiles, and I was thrown back in my chair, ears ringing and slightly stunned myself.

'What the hell was that?'

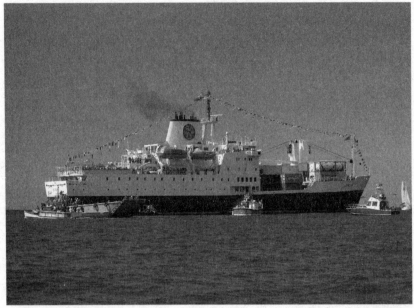

RMS *St Helena* in full regalia with flotilla preparing for her last voyage

I had most certainly killed the plank, also the carpet beneath, and furthermore dug a crater in the concrete floor that would have done justice to the lunar surface.

'Oh no. Ken – look!'

Ken had a glazed, even trancelike expression. I held up the gun, the bolt now protruding from the muzzle, its end, a sharpened cylinder of steel, splayed open like a cartoon exploding cigar.

I had been entrusted with the RMS's antique stun gun, and I had destroyed it. I was mortified. I had failed to take into account that this was an old design.

'Ken, the kickback is vicious. There can't be any cushions in this gun.' The modern stun gun has a set of Polo-shaped rubber cushions stacked along the internal section of the bolt, taking up the impetus and bringing the bolt to a relatively comfortable halt. That was evidently a modern refinement and a good one. This stun gun was more like a blunderbuss. 'Now what do I do?'

Mr Fixit was already on the case. 'Don't worry, Joe. I'll take it down to Theodore at the government garage.' Theodore was a skilled metalworker and had only recently machined a thread into an orthopaedic pin so that I could fix a particularly tricky femoral fracture. 'I'm sure he can lathe off the end and give it a new edge. As for the floor and carpet, we'll, um... I think we'll just cover it up,' he added hastily.

HAIRY SHEEP

The sheep on St Helena were steeped in the genetics of colonial influence: woolly European breeds – hardly suited to a tropical island. Breeds such as the Cheviot, a northern hill sheep; the Romney Marsh, a hardy bog sheep; and even the Swaledale, a Yorkshire Dales sheep, surely brought on the whim of a homesick Yorkshireman.

The great woollen mills of Britain were designed to clothe the Empire, uniform her armies, carpet her living rooms and hallways, and for this, sheep breeds were developed that grew thick, heavy fleeces; leather and meat were secondary products. St Helena's beautiful, steep upland pastures are unfit for cultivation but merit stewardship, and sheep are excellent custodians of the rampant sward. But St Helena has no use for their wool, and every year the ageing and arthritic sheep-owning farmers would hand shear the flocks, backbreaking toil, and dump the wool outside the sheep pens, where it would be left to rot and drift in the wind like persistent dirty snow.

Worse, far worse, it was a revelation for me to discover that in the tropics a heavy rain shower followed by a blast of sun could quickly brew up the Devil's own potion: blowfly myiasis. Flystrike. The 'blue buzzers' home in and lay their eggs, and within days legions of maggots eat the sheep alive, pouring out digestive enzymes and sucking in the juices to nourish their staggeringly fast rate of growth.

Maggots have their role, and it's an important one. We need them, and not just as groundbait for old men fishing for eels on muddy canals. They neatly and efficiently dispose of and recycle the dead. But to be eaten alive, morsel by tiny morsel, is a torture that no animal should endure. Flystrike is terrible for sheep and expensive for farmers.

This was where the hair sheep came in.

I'd checked out all the hair breeds, such as the Katahdin and the Barbados Blackbelly, and concluded that the Dorper was the most tried and tested version. A legendary Saint, Skipper, had tried once before with crossbreds brought in from Ascension but the experiment had not been completely successful. We needed purebreds.

The Dorper is a South African breed, an easy-care, prolific lamber expressly designed to survive in harsh conditions. South African breeders skilfully combined the characteristics of two diametrically opposed breeds: the Dorset Horn, English with a lovely temperament and the added bonus that, unlike other breeds, it cycles all year round, allowing three crops of lambs every two years; and the Persian Blackhead, a hairy Middle Eastern breed, goat-like both in its appearance and toughness. The coarse hair coat resists flystrike, and sheds annually: 'self-shearing', as the breeders like to say. It has the added advantage of not covering the crotch and underbelly, avoiding the problem of dags – shitty dreadlocks that attract flies – and the need to dock tails.

Put the two breeds' characteristics together in one neat sheepy package and you have an animal that is a non-selective grazer, hardier in marginal conditions, a placid, easy lamber with good mothering abilities and a high twinning rate, and only needs a tidy with the sheep shears – although admittedly the hair challenges the blades. Fewer hours tending, higher survival rate, heavier lambs, and plumper mutton stews.

In defiance of my own strongly held principles of biosecurity, I wanted to import live pedigrees to kickstart the Dorperisation of the local sheep. Live animals are, naturally, Noah's arks for microbes. For this reason, I favoured importation from the UK rather than from South Africa, which can sometimes be lacking in terms of checks and certification. I planned to have every parasite wiped from my Dorpers' bodies and their blood and faeces tested to the boondocks and beyond.

Fortunately, I found that the British Dorper Sheep Society comprised a bunch of enthusiasts who loved a novel project and were led by an energetic chairman, Andrew Baker. Months of toing and froing ensued, poring over pedigrees to avoid incestuously close offspring, drafting export health certificates, negotiating prices and payments, researching and defining the best testing protocol, and fine-tuning the logistics, even down to measuring the ventilation rate in the RMS's livestock pen with the help of the ship's engineer, and calculating the legal requirement for bales of hay enshrined in EU legislation should the ship be left helpless and drifting. And, of course, teaching Captain Andrew how to kill sheep.

The distillation of all these endeavours was seven rams and four ewes from separate families, drawn from eight Society members scattered between Wales, northern England, and the West Country. The sheep would be quarantined for several weeks, tested, and then certified as fit to travel, whereupon four of the farmers would collect the cargo and weave their separate ways down to the port in Dorset on departure day. I had spent thousands of pounds of government money in advance payments to set it all up. It was, I flattered myself, an elegant plan in which I had covered all eventualities.

I hadn't.

It only takes a pin prick to burst a balloon, no matter how pretty that balloon may be.

ASCENSION ISLAND

The 800-mile three-day trip up to Ascension was a workers' voyage; Saints returning to Ascension after a break at home. The atmosphere was tense, even oppressive, and I doubted my wisdom in choosing to go the whole sixteen days to the UK.

There is no citizenship on Ascension. The rule is: no job, no can stay. But the sister island to St Helena has always provided Saints with remunerative employment. It is a strategic military base and listening post, where the RAF rubs shoulders with the USAF, an island of frozen, jagged lava flows, of ash pits, barren craters and hillocks of pumice, in total contrast to the fortress cliffs and green-clad peaks of St Helena. No wonder that they used jokingly to call St Helena 'The Old Rock' and Ascension 'The Cinder'. But it also has glorious beaches of soft white sand, shiny red and yellow land crabs that look moulded in plastic, turtle nesting sites by the gazillion and, strangest of all amid this volcanic devastation, Green Mountain, a lush central peak with its own microclimate. It is the world's first ever example of terra-forming, metamorphosised by colonial naturalists broadcasting handfuls of exotic seeds to see if they would germinate. Darwin himself is said to have sprinkled a few.

I had one week before the return of the RMS to fulfil my duties. The island always tickled my imagination with its strange marrying of various entities, the angle-iron armies of tall aerials

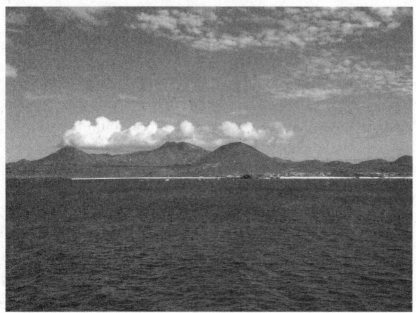

Ascension viewed from the RMS, with
Green Mountain visible in the centre

immobilised by taut networks of cables like stick insects in a web, alongside the ornate and colourful architecture of Georgetown baking under a relentless equatorial sun.

Caz Yon, the European Space Agency's tracking station operator, had a secondary role as a paravet caring for the island's pets, wild donkeys and feral sheep, which she did with great care and competence. She took me under her wing, and I worked my way through consultations, operations and house visits, dispensing advice and medications to the expat community. My stint duly done, I relaxed for a few days with walks along the old military lookout paths threaded around and through the top of Green Mountain, and spectacular dives with Galapagos sharks in the lee of Boatswain Bird Island.

Eventually the friendly mustard funnel and crisp blue hull of the RMS *St Helena* hove into view and she dropped anchor in

Clarence Bay. I boarded to find the atmosphere on board wholly transformed. This was a holiday ship: pre-prandial cocktail parties, the officers mingling in full rig; deck cricket, whacking hempen 'monkey's fists' into loosely strung nets (overboard and your score is wiped); 'gin for Jesus' with the captain after Sunday service (I'm sure, with His water-to-wine feat fully documented, He would have grudgingly approved); 'crossing the line' hilarity as the equator was pierced, Neptune's mermaids smothering novitiates in baked beans and cold spaghetti before flinging them into the pool; endless quizzes, movies and games; and prodigal quantities of food and drink. Plus, all the time in the world to chill and read a book while the bow cleaved the waves and the sea hissed along the keel. A former crew member, Matt Joshua, even led a group of us dressed as pirates in a mock storming of the bridge, where we were received by the captain with great bonhomie and no brandishing of the apocryphal handgun. I couldn't imagine any other ship where this would have been tolerated as a jolly jape, although the skull-and-crossbones bicorne hats may have been the giveaway.

Governor Gurr was on board and the building of the St Helena Airport was a hot topic, so he requested a slight deviation in the vessel's course: past the eastern shore of Madeira to view the famous stilted airport. The precipitous volcanic topography of Madeira has much in common with St Helena, but on a more colossal scale. They had been forced to wrestle with the same problem: where do you put a flat, one-and-three-quarter-mile-long airstrip in a landscape that denies the horizontal? Their answer was to build a coastal airport on pillars.

Captain Rodney veered the RMS towards the Madeiran coast and the passengers lined the rails, Governor Gurr holding forth on the value of building an airport. The white columns shone in the sunlight like an elongated Parthenon, and oohs and aahs rippled through the onlookers as a jet flew across the scene then banked hard around through 180° to drop abruptly onto the raised platform beneath a soaring hillside crowded with houses.

'That,' shouted the Governor, ever the showman and stabbing a finger at the whole of Madeira as if piercing a sausage, 'is what we need!'

The days trickled by. Waistlines expanded, the sea turned slowly from blue to grey, the air cooled, the clouds gathered and the return to reality dawned on us, until at last we entered the busy approaches to the English Channel. Finally we rounded Portland Bill to dock at the old naval base.

Teeny was there to meet me and we went back to my petite, brick-and-slate cottage in its pretty rural village enfolded within the chalk downland of Hampshire. I felt a deep sense of calm with six weeks of unencumbered holiday to enjoy. All I had was the minor task of loading my sheep and chickens in ten days' time when the ship was ready to sail back to St Helena. Meanwhile, the ship was offloading and backloading cargoes, changing crews and captains, having her rust spots chipped and sanded, her gantries repainted, engines serviced, carpets shampooed, even her bell burnished, until she was satisfactorily shipshape and Bristol fashion. And, as a UK-registered vessel, all her certifications and registrations renewed.

Including her Animal Transporter Authorisation.

The pin was fast approaching my beautiful balloon.

THE PIN PRICK

It was the eve of the RMS's departure. Across the country, farmers were readying their vehicles and vets were conducting their final examinations and certifications. All my animals were poised ready for the off.

I had been trying to phone the Chief Officer, Peter Milton, to check all was well but he had been deeply occupied by recertifying the ship with the Maritime Coastal Agency and had switched off his mobile. I had no doubt he would have contacted me if there were any problems, and I had kept in touch with all other parties. There was nothing to worry about.

The phone rang. It was one of the vets.

'I was just doing final certification for Rob Grinall's sheep,' he said, 'but I received a message from the AHVLA to say they're not going.'

The AHVLA: the Animal Health and Veterinary Laboratories Agency, an executive branch of the ministry of agriculture. This was a cataclysmic statement.

'Not going? No – I'm sure there's some mistake. They've passed all their tests. Why would the AHVLA say that?'

'I'm not sure exactly,' he went on. 'Some balls up with the ship's licence to carry animals.'

I was stunned. 'But... but I've heard nothing. The ship's leaving tomorrow, for goodness' sake.'

'Sorry, but that's the message.'

My mind was racing with possibilities. There were only a few hours left before the livestock trailers began their long overnight journeys to the south coast. A failure of gargantuan proportions loomed. 'Look, do me a favour,' I urged, thinking on the hoof. 'Could you fill in the certificate anyway as the sheep have satisfied all the criteria, and I'll see what I can do to sort this out? Please tell Rob to carry on as planned and I'll phone him later.' It was a hideous gamble.

'Sure. No problem my end. And good luck. I think you'll need it.'

It was already approaching eight p.m., dangerously late for remedial action. I knew the EU animal transport legislation inside out, and it was true that the RMS didn't have things such as secondary alarms in the wheelhouse for a failure of the water, lighting or ventilation, but we had something better: vigilance and clipboards, watch in, watch out. The ministry knew this and had given us derogations. Something else had gone wrong.

I dialled the number for the shipping agent, who I knew was down at the dock. We had an email association but had rarely met face to face.

'Jim, what's the issue with the sheep? I've just been informed they can't board.'

'That's right. No go, I'm afraid.'

'Really? Why's that? I thought we had everything in order.'

'They examined the livestock pen and were happy with most of it. Just a few minor bits and pieces like protruding edges, old mesh, paint and so on, but the crew quickly fixed those. However, they didn't like the troughs.'

'The troughs? What about the troughs?'

'They were wood. They don't like wood. It's unhygienic. So the Chief Officer had them ripped out and stainless-steel replacements welded in the dockyard. Very good they are too.'

'So why are the troughs still a problem? Can't they fit them?'

'No, they're fitted all right. But the ship was then meant to email photos to AHVLA to prove that all the improvements had been made. Unfortunately, though, the ship's link has gone down.'

'What?' I could feel frustration building up inside me. 'Do you mean to say that it's all down to a few photos?'

'That's right.'

'Did no one have the nous to put them on a USB stick and go to an internet café – or even the police station? Or anyone... anyone...' I repeated emphatically, my voice getting louder, '...with a computer? I've been sitting here for the past ten days. Why has no one contacted me about this? I'm the bloody vet! We've just a few hours before departure... I have farmers and vets all over the country... livestock trailers... chickens... I've spent thousands—'

'Well, I'm sorry,' he cut in icily, 'but anyway it's too late now. Nothing to be done.' I could hear that he cared not a bean for my sheep and chickens. He was ready for a nice meal, a glass or two and a comfy bed. 'It's been a long day, and I'm off to my hotel. Bye.' And the accursed man hung up.

It was one of those theatrical moments when I stood limply for a moment staring blindly at the receiver. But in a way he was right: the offices of the AHVLA were closed, and the chance of salvaging the situation was as likely as finding a diamond in a cesspit.

The AHVLA. They had a twenty-four-hour emergency service. I delved around in phone numbers until I came up with a contact and dialled my way through a few answerphones. Eventually, by some miracle, I found a living vet.

'Ah yes,' said Nicola Hirst, a hint of irritation in her voice. 'I've been fully apprised of the situation. You are forbidden to load the sheep or the chickens, and we'll be there to make sure you don't. All we wanted was photographic proof. Not much to ask for really, is it? But no – nothing.'

She sounded hard, but at the same time reasonable. It was time to go vet to vet. I heartily agreed with her mildly expressed annoyance, explained why they had failed, expounded on my sheer exasperation that no one had had the gumption to find an outside internet connection, then played a most melodic violin extemporising on how the sheep were to transform the island's agriculture, condition the landscape, put food in islanders' mouths and money in their pockets. And that this was the RMS's last scheduled journey to the UK for a very long time. I even added a little travelogue about St Helena and recommended a visit.

'OK,' she sighed. I could hear her thawing around the edges. 'Get me these wretched photos.'

Always leave the bad news until last. 'I have to tell you, though, that I'm seventy miles from Portland. There and back plus shenanigans on board, it's going to be at least four hours. Then I need to upload the photos and email them to you. That puts us at two or three in the morning. I'm so sorry.'

A slight hesitation and maybe a suppressed groan, then the angel at the other end replied: 'I'll wait up. But I'll give you my mobile. Phone me from the ship and we'll go through my checklist to make sure all the pictures are there. Otherwise, I can't clear you, and I have the last say.'

Now the next problem: to advise the ship. I phoned the shipping agent again, but his mobile was off. So too, as ever, was Peter Milton's. I slammed the receiver down. 'Oh, that's bloody fantastic!'

'What now?' Teeny was watching the events unfold with shared anxiety.

'The damn agent's switched off his phone and I have absolutely no way of contacting the ship. I'm just going to have to drive down there and chance it.'

I bit the bullet and rang around the farmers with the message 'Go, go, go' and having initiated the mass launching of live-stock trailers, slumped against the wall by the telephone, heart pounding, completely hyped up on adrenaline. The first out would be John Rowlands, a charming farmer from the Welsh

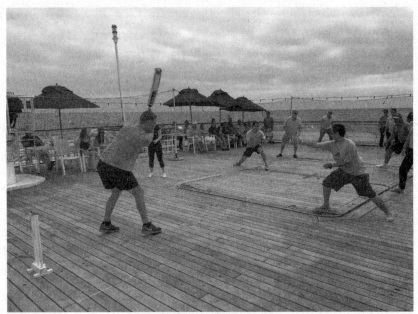

Deck cricket aboard RMS *St Helena*

island of Anglesey, and I imagined his trailer rumbling across the Menai Straits bridge. 'Teeny, if I sort this out, I'll deserve a bloody medal. And if I don't, it's going to be pandemonium. I'll be hung, drawn and quartered.' I could see a chaotic dockside crammed with cackling chickens and bleating sheep, and irate farmers waving calloused fists.

'You'll sort it,' she replied, with a confidence I didn't share. 'Here.' She threw a steaming omelette in my direction. 'Eat or you'll never make it. And drive carefully.'

Easier said than done.

Traffic was light but the weather gods were in on the joke and threw down a blanket of thick coastal fog. At first I made good time, speeding along and dodging speed cameras with just a slight pang of guilt, but then the fog intensified and my progress was reduced to an achingly slow crawl. Finally, I pulled into the docks.

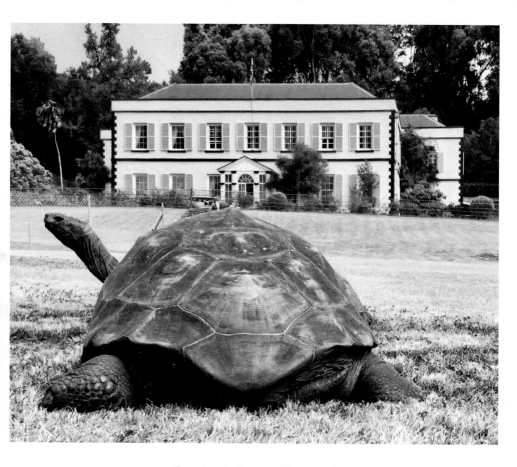

ABOVE: Jonathan in front of Plantation House.
BELOW: Joe feeding Jonathan. *Both photos by Teeny Lucy.*

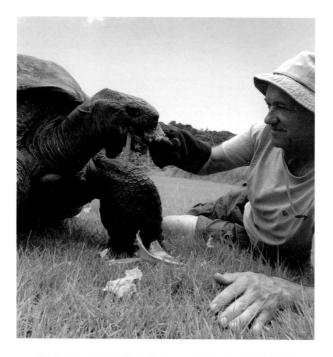

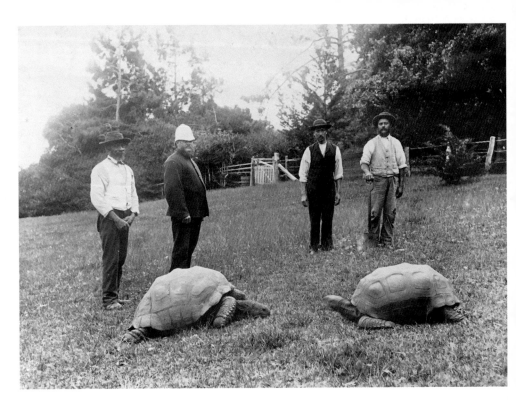

ABOVE: Jonathan (left) in the late 1800s with Saints (islanders). *Image by Alexander Lee Innes.*
BELOW: The Butcher's Grave in Plantation Forest.

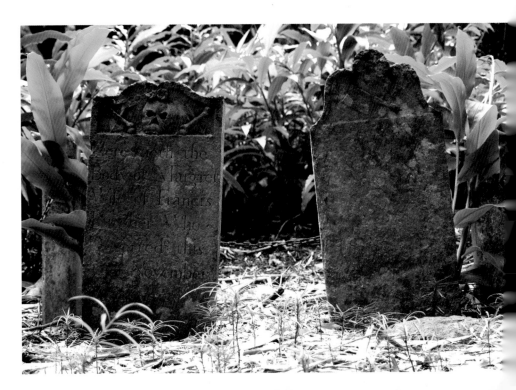

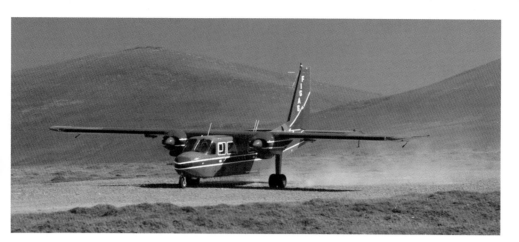

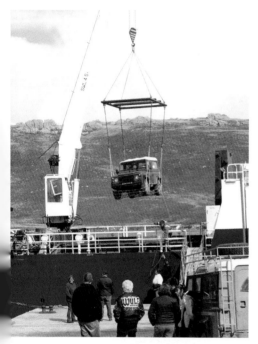

TOP: A FIGAS Islander aircraft coming in to land. CENTER: Crossing to West Falkland—my Landie being offloaded at Port Howard. BOTTOM: A typical Falkland landing strip at Bleaker Island.

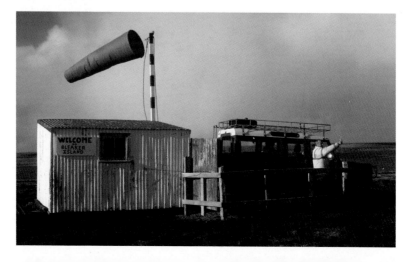

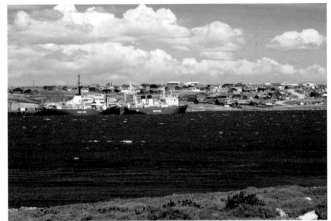

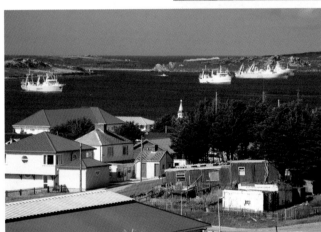

TOP: Fishery patrol vessels moored at Stanley, viewed from across the harbor.
CENTER: Fishing vessels in Stanley Harbor.
BOTTOM: Gentoo penguins at King George Bay, West Falkland.

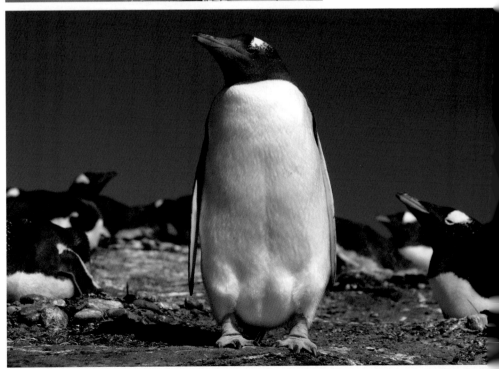

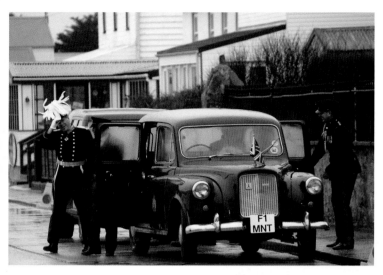

TOP: The Falkland Islands governor in full ceremonial dress arrives for the Liberation Day service. CENTER: Falkland Islands Liberation Day ceremonies. BOTTOM: One of the many different architectural styles of Stanley. This one is a home converted from a Nissan hut.

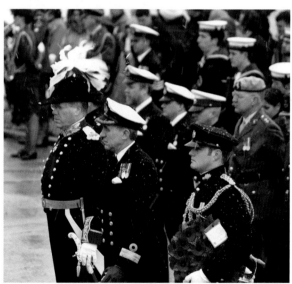

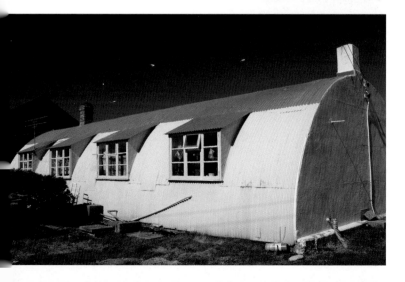

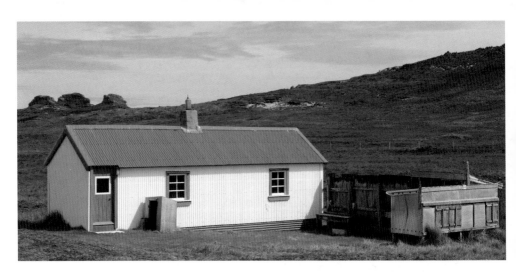

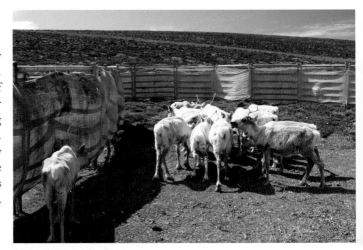

TOP: The shepherd's shanty at Three Crowns, Albemarle. CENTER: The herd of depleted reindeer inside our makeshift pen, awaiting transfer to Albemarle. BOTTOM: Teeny Lucy and our New Year's Eve feast inside the shepherd's shanty at Three Crowns.

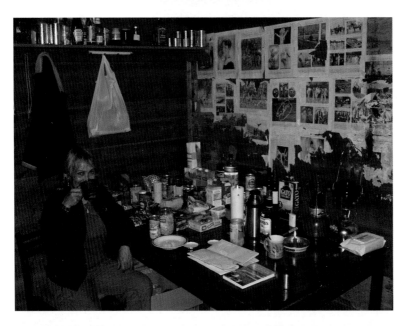

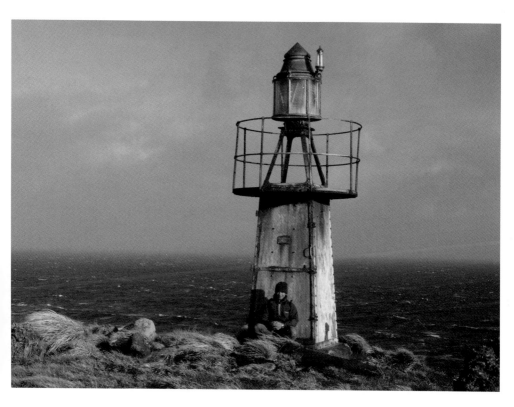

ABOVE: The author at the Cape Meredith beacon.
BELOW: A rejuvenated reindeer feeding at Albemarle, New Year's Day.

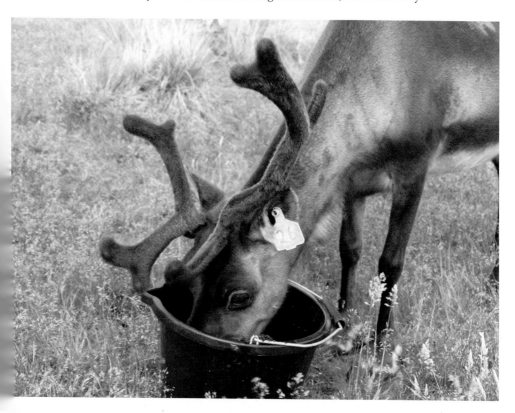

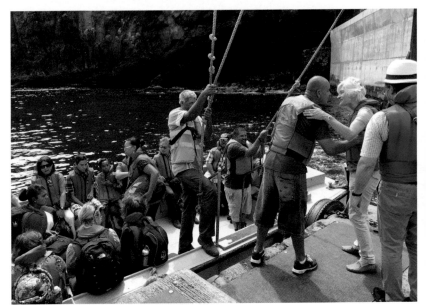

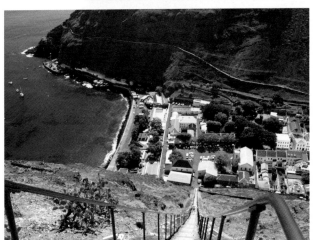

TOP: Landing and entering St. Helena by rope from the Steps.
CENTER: Jamestown seen from the top of the 699 thigh-bruising steps of Jacob's Ladder.
BOTTOM: Veterinary assistant Rico Williams at our clinic.

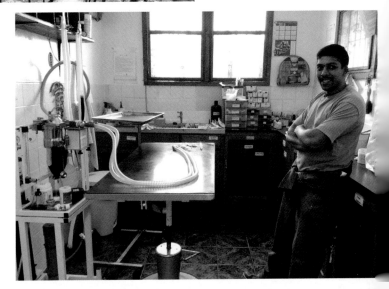

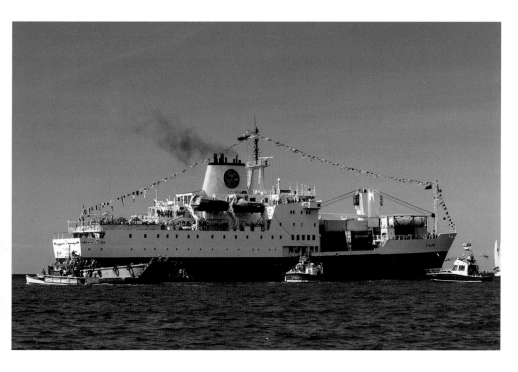

ABOVE: The RMS *St. Helena* in full regalia with flotilla preparing for her last voyage. BELOW: Ascension Island viewed from the RMS *St. Helena*, with Green Mountain—the first example of terraforming—visible in the center.

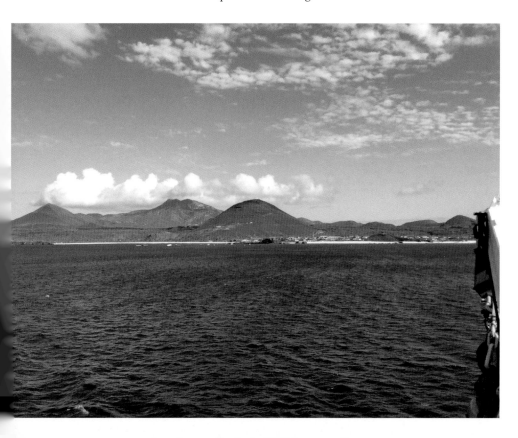

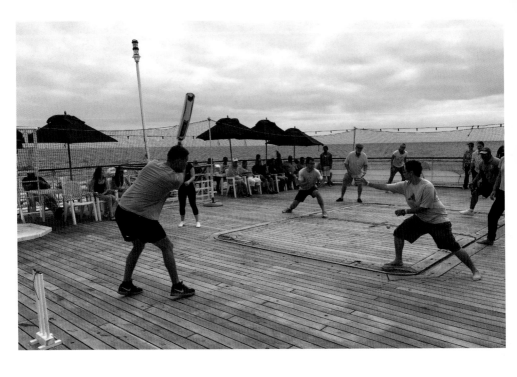

ABOVE: Deck cricket aboard the RMS *St. Helena*.
BELOW: A Dorper ram safely ensconced among the flock at Botley's Ley.

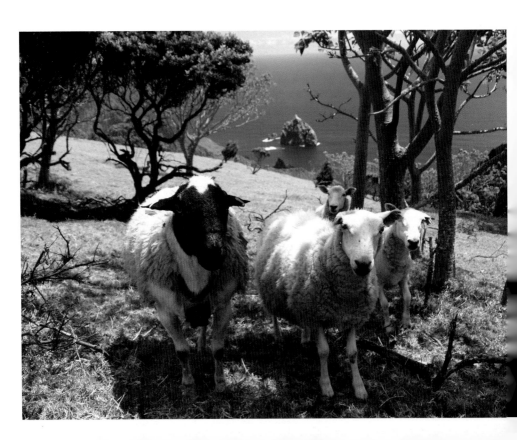

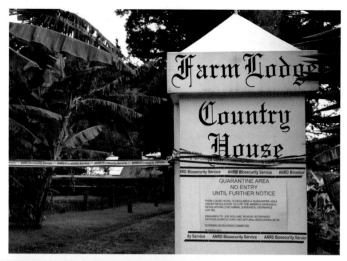

TOP: Farm Lodge goes into quarantine to prevent the spread of fowl cholera. CENTER: Mustering the doomed ducks for humane euthanasia. BOTTOM: St. Mary's Church, Georgetown, Ascension Island.

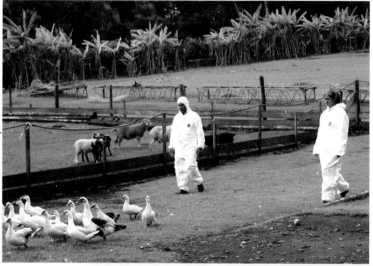

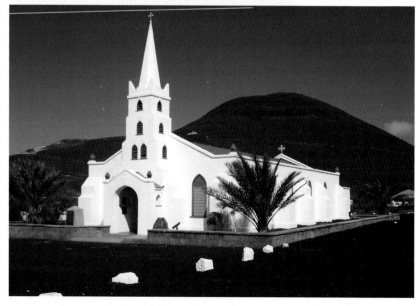

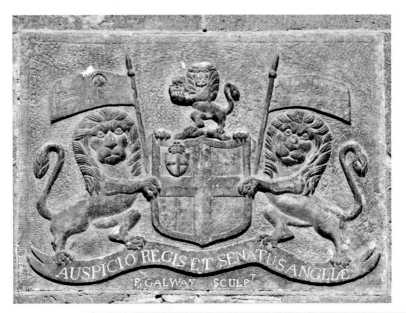

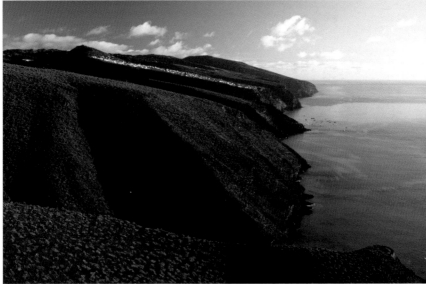

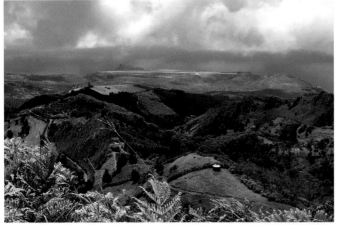

TOP: The East India Company coat of arms with the motto: "By command of the King and Parliament of England." CENTER: Looking toward Jamestown from Sugar Loaf. BOTTOM: The newly constructed St. Helena airport, its runway visible on the horizon.

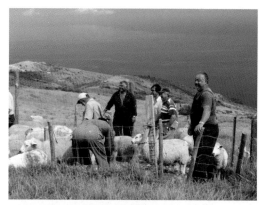

TOP: The sheep pound on St. Helena at Man and Horse with Gary Stevens, Trevor Glass, and others. CENTER: The Settlement on Tristan, with the black lava flows of the 1961 eruption visible to the left. BOTTOM: The Potato Patches on Tristan.

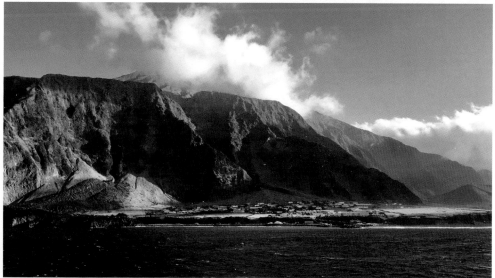

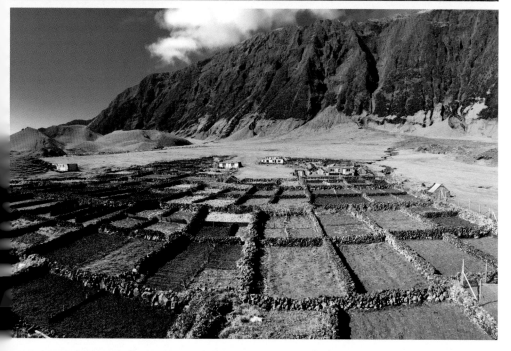

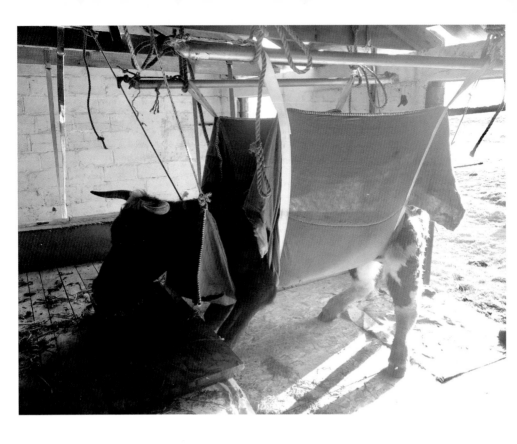

ABOVE: One of Tristan's downer cows recuperating in the sling.
BELOW: Counting rockhopper penguins on Middle Island, Nightingale, Tristan da Cunha.

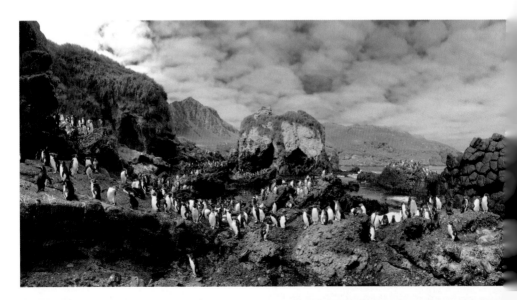

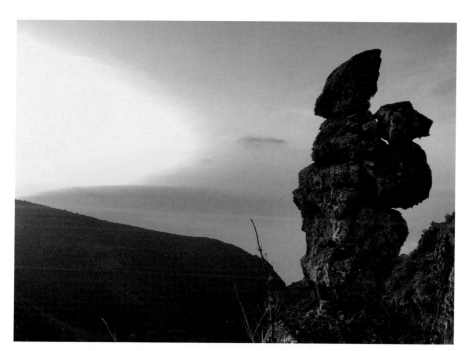

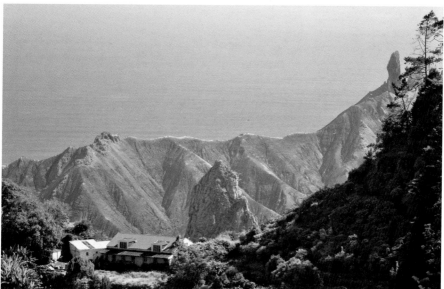

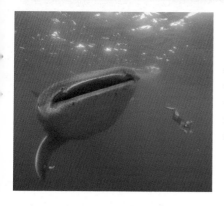

TOP: The Friar. CENTER: A view of ridges with Lot (foreground) and Lot's Wife (on the farther ridge) from Mount Pleasant. BOTTOM: Me freediving with a whale shark off St. Helena. *Photo by Dr. Attila Frigyesi.*

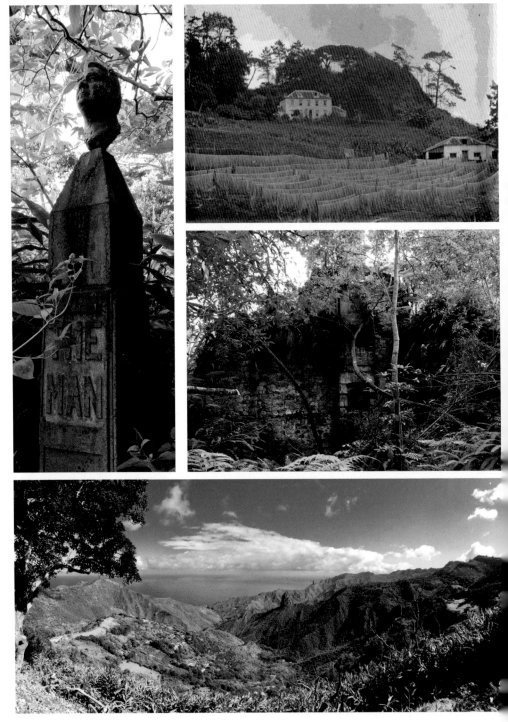

TOP LEFT: Former owner Tony Thornton's statue erected by him to himself on the grounds of Rose Cottage. TOP RIGHT: Rose Cottage and her flax farm in the late nineteenth century. *Image by Thomas Jackson.* CENTER RIGHT: Rose Cottage as she is now. BOTTOM: The view from Rose Cottage.

It was a dank and inky night, lit only by the muted glow of security lights. Everything was dripping with condensation, all sound stifled by the fog. I parked my car and walked up to a kiosk by a barrier, the hull of the RMS just visible beyond. Inside the kiosk, a grandfatherly old man with a grizzled moustache and a peaked cap was perched on a chair, half buried in a thick, navy-blue overcoat.

'Oh hullo. What can I be doing you for?' he asked, quite perkily for the hour.

I pulled out my passport to prove who I was and pleaded my case. A broad smile slowly rippled his cheeks. 'Sheep, eh? Well, well, well. And I thought I'd heard it all.' He thumbed through my passport with an appraising eye, tickled with amusement. 'Let's see what we can do,' he said pleasantly, and reached for the two-way radio. 'Security to bridge, security to bridge. I have a young chap here to see you about some sheep. Name's Hollins. Over.'

'Hollins? The vet? OK, let him board. Over.'

A crewman met me at the gangway and escorted me up to the officers' cabins. It was after midnight, the graveyard watch, and the ship was bedded down for the night, cloaked in silence with minimal lighting, but all buffed and ready to burst into the hustle and bustle of departure day. 'The Old Man's not aboard yet,' said the crewman, referring to Captain Andrew in the traditional manner, 'so you'll have to see the Chief Officer. But I warn you... he's fast asleep and won't be happy.'

He wasn't. He was apoplectic. Peter Milton stood in his cabin door with a towel around his waist and a face of fury. 'What the bloody hell are you doing here?' he exploded, his eyes blazing as he ran his hand through his dishevelled hair. 'What time do you call this? Don't you know we've a ship to run?'

'The sheep...'

'Sheep? I couldn't give a shit about your fucking sheep.'

I'd had enough. 'Peter! I've just driven seventy miles far too fast in the fog to get here, I've another seventy to go back, I've got a ministry vet waiting up for me on the end of a phone, and I've pissed off the shipping agent. All this because you didn't keep me in the loop and switched off your mobile. You think I'm happy about that? I'm thoroughly hacked off. Why the hell didn't you contact me?'

'Give him the damn pictures,' he growled, and slammed his cabin door.

I stood for a moment, suitably chastened and spittle flecked. The crewman gave me a friendly nudge. 'Don't mind Peter,' he grinned. 'He's just a tad stressed.'

Up on the bridge, the officer of the watch plugged in my USB stick and uploaded the pictures while we chatted amiably. I phoned Nicola Hirst at the AHVLA and went through her checklist, ironed out a few niggles, then grabbed the stick and headed back out into the fog. Another long drive, this time not quite as frenetic, and I parked up by my cottage just before two a.m. I prayed that my internet was working and uploaded the pictures. Minutes later the phone rang. It was the ever-patient Nicola.

'You're all good,' she said sleepily. 'I'm going to stand down my team. I'll send you a formal email, but you're free to load your sheep. And I hope it goes well.'

'I can't thank you enough.' Her words were balm to the soul. Humiliation, rancour and agricultural fisticuffs on the dockside narrowly avoided.

But there's no rest for the wicked – or innocent sheep farmers come to that. Mine were wending their way down through the country, and it was almost time for me to wend my way once more down to Portland. A reviving cup of tea, a couple of hours kip fully dressed on the sofa, and then yet again I drove off into the dreary night, but this time at a leisurely pace, humming along to the ramblings of the early morning DJs.

At eight a.m., the crew were readying the ship to receive passengers, the derrick frantically loading final items of cargo. I heard the familiar rumble of a livestock trailer and turned to see John Rowlands in a Range Rover slaloming his way between the stevedores and crates scattered along the wharf. He rolled to a halt, all the way from Anglesey. First out and first in.

'John! What a pleasure. We meet at last.' I grasped his gnarly hand and shook it vigorously. John was a delight to talk to, an archetypal Welsh sheep farmer and, typical of his hard-working tribe, showed not one iota of fatigue from his long journey.

'Come and see your rams. I've got you a pair of beauties.'

I peered through the slats of his livestock trailer.

'That's Pwyll, which means Caution, but he's as soft as a lamb. And that's Ffa Pob – Baked Beans. I named him after breakfast one day.'

In the rear section of the trailer two stout, young rams, black heads and white hairy bodies, eyed us calmly. They were well handled and looked no worse for their journey. With his rare, Labrador-like temperament, Pwyll would rapidly become a favourite back on St Helena, though because of his unusually broad skull and heavy, muscular body, my veterinary team switched his name to Samson. Samson went on to woo many Delilahs and fill the hills with his babies.

Soon all four trailers were assembled on the dock, along with my supplies: ten bales of straw, twenty-four bales of hay and ten bags of sheep nuts. A fifth trailer rolled in carrying the sixty

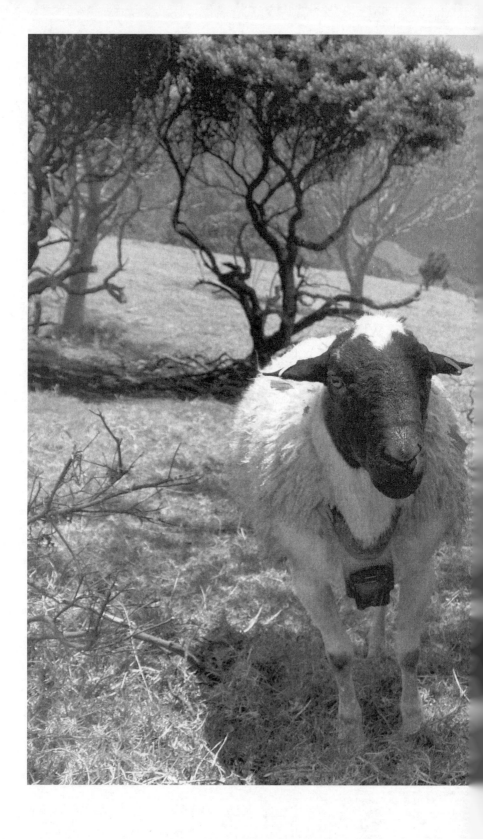

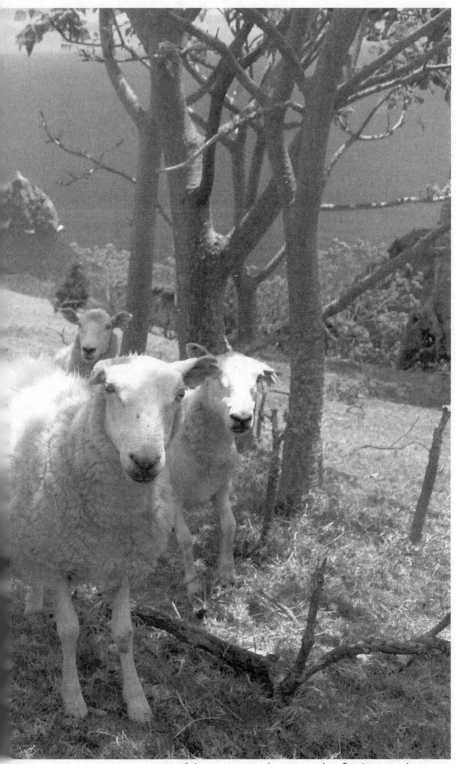
A Dorper ram safely ensconced among the flock at Botleys Ley

point-of-lay Lohmann Brown chickens to fill our government incubators with eggs and the islanders' plates with scramble. The farmers chatted away enthusiastically about Dorpers and all things farming in a harmonious orchestration of West Country burr, Welsh singsong and northern inflection, while the local press buzzed around taking photos, getting John to hug up his two rams and primping the angle of his cloth cap against the backdrop of the RMS's distinctive funnel. There was hearty laughter, the clucking of hens, an occasional baa, and the bustle of a busy quay: a country-fair ambience that filled my soul with pleasure – and not a little relief.

I had done it. And not one fist raised in anger.

A hand rested briefly on my shoulder, and I looked round to see Chief Officer Peter Milton. 'Joe, sorry about last night. We've just been so hectic, what with the MCA poking their noses into everything. But well done. Mission accomplished, eh?'

An apology from a merchant seaman is a rare thing. 'Peter, no problem at all,' I replied, patting his left arm. 'Water off a seal's back.' I knew him to be sound, and frankly, after a profoundly stressful night spent plucking victory from the jaws of defeat, I couldn't care less.

My attention was caught by a suited figure clutching a brief-case and walking hesitantly through the dockside farmyard with a look of bewilderment. It was Jim, the agent. For a moment our eyes locked and he all too quickly broke away and scuttled up the gangplank. Not even a paltry word of acknowledgement passed his miserly lips. I stared at his receding back with the eyes of an assassin. I wondered how well he could swim and how long the jail sentence would be.

I supervised the loading, made sure the sheep and poultry were strawed down and settled in their pens, gave the shipboard doctor a veterinary kit and a brief guide I'd compiled on dose rates and common sheep ailments, then massacred a jug of coffee and a stack of toast in the ship's mess. A final key person loomed into view. The Old Man was aboard.

'I hear congratulations are in order, Joe. I gather you had a bit of a night of it.' Captain Andrew was immaculately uniformed, ready to receive and impress his passengers, and as charming and polite as always. 'I nearly lost my chance to try out the old blunderbuss.'

'Don't jest!' We both laughed anyway.

He shook my hand. 'Duties to attend to. See you back on the island.'

I finished my coffee, brushed away the crumbs of toast, stretched back and relaxed. Time for some well-earned holiday at last. I just had to hope the old blunderbuss stayed firmly locked away in the captain's safe, alongside the apocryphal handgun.

It did.

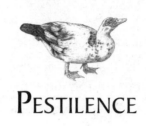

PESTILENCE

故曰知彼知己百戰不殆
不知彼而知己一勝一負
不知彼不知己每戰必殆

If you know the enemy and know yourself, you
need not fear the result of a hundred battles
If you know yourself but not the enemy, for every
victory gained you will also suffer defeat
If you know neither the enemy nor yourself,
you will succumb in every battle

孫子 General Sun Tzu, *The Art of War*, fifth century BCE

A SEADOG CALLS

It began innocuously enough, more a pest than a plague. The
plague was to come.

'Joe, I've a present for you.' Steve Biggs, a salty seadog with
a weather-beaten face and an enviable drift of pure white hair,
stood outside the surgery dangling a brace of very dead ducks
from his right hand. 'I've lost a couple of others too.'

A Saint couple is not a couple.

'Biggsy, is that a British couple, a Saint couple, or a nice
couple?' I asked, adding the third local elaboration.

'Oh yes.' He laughed. 'I see what you mean. Actually, a nice
couple. Ten or twelve.'

I was taken aback. 'Oh, damn. That's not right. I'll post-mortem these and see what we can find out.'

I've extolled the virtues of post-mortems before, but there's no getting away from it: all the medical imaging in the world can't compete against a forensic dissection of the victim for providing answers. But at first the two Muscovy ducks – known locally as Scobies – posed more questions than they supplied answers.

I phoned Steve with the results. 'Steve, it's bloody odd, and something I've never seen before. Their livers were swollen and covered in small white spots, and there was a pericarditis – an inflammation around the heart – with extensive haemorrhages into the heart muscle. No doubt why they died, just not sure what from.'

'I see.' Steve sounded anxious. 'The thing is, Joe, it's getting worse. I was walking through them earlier this afternoon and one keeled over and dropped dead at my feet.'

'Dropped dead? Steve, how many ducks do you have?'

'About a hundred and ten, all Scobies, Khaki Campbells and their crosses. And then, of course, there are the guinea fowl and the chickens, but they seem unaffected.'

Alarm bells were jangling. This had all the elements of a disease outbreak, but one with significant pathogenicity. It was my turn to be anxious. Anxious about extinction.

Before the advent of man on St Helena, before João da Nova planted his espadrilles on her gritty shores in 1502 and we ravaged the countryside and plundered the island's resources, there were several endemic bird species, including a giant hoopoe, which would have been tourism gold for drawing in the flocks of migratory twitchers. Now there is only one: *Charadrius sanctaehe-lenae*, the iconic wirebird, as depicted on the island's coat of arms (recently updated to make it look less like a bedraggled seagull).

St Helena has been an island of extinctions. Birds, arthropods and plants galore that took millions of years to evolve have been consigned to complete and eternal oblivion in just five hundred. Still, somehow, on land and in sea, the island holds one third of endemic species to be found on all British territory, including the UK.

When I first arrived on the island, wirebird numbers were plunging. All the predictions and extrapolations indicated that the species would finally succumb and become another dismal entry on that shameful list within a mere ten years. Ten years! Drastic action had to be taken. There followed a concerted effort between different agencies to salvage the species through the trapping and humane euthanasia of its main predator: the feral cat. Which is where I came in. We launched the compulsory microchipping of pet cats, cheap neutering and a high-welfare system of euthanasia for ferals that proceeded with a triple-mix general anaesthetic – allowing a scan for a microchip – followed by the *coup de grâce*, a lethal injection. Fortunately, pet cats sit sedately in a trap and miaow, whereas feral cats hiss and spit and weave back and forth like caged pumas, behaviours that virtually eliminate the terrible mishap of euthanising someone's beloved Tibby.

This was not anti-cat. Cats do what cats are designed to do; they are superlative hunters and fascinating animals. The fault lay with humans releasing them into a habitat they had no right to be in. Sad though it all was, I knew that we were acting as ethically as possible. And the reward has been an undeniable upturn in wirebird numbers, dragging them back from the brutal brink of extinction.

In addition to the wirebird, St Helena has extensive seabird colonies, from the ethereal, pure-white fairy terns that nest high in the forests carrying bait fish to their young, and the tiny

Madeiran storm petrels that clip the cresting waves like oceanic darts, to the masked boobies and the long-tailed tropic birds that sail along the cliffs and paint the coastal ridges with guano.

I simply couldn't stand by and witness the unleashing of an avian epidemic.

'Steve, I'm coming over.'

THE MURDEROUS DUMBBELL

Steve was a true Devonian, born to the briny then sent into the merchant navy by his father to follow the family tradition. Eventually he served as purser on the RMS and there met his partner Maureen Jonas, one of the stewardesses and a dyed-in-the-wool Saint. When they both finally hung up their windcheaters and came ashore, they bought Farm Lodge, a dilapidated seventeenth-century East India Company planter's house set in ten sloping acres and flanked by a cliff. Through sheer unending diligence, they transformed it into a shining pearl.

It is both a farm and a country hotel. It is also a coffee plantation and grows one of the finest and most expensive coffees in the world, the green-tipped Bourbon Arabica, traded – or perhaps purloined – from the port city of Mocha in Yemen back in 1733, and currently for sale in Harrods of London at a humble £600 per kilo.

Why? Because the green-tipped Bourbon Arabica is nature's true, original, unhybridised coffee, enriched by volcanic soils, watered by the distilled vapours of the South Atlantic, and ripened in the sweet, unpolluted airs of remote insularity. If I wax on about its virtues, it is because every visit ended with a French press of this luxurious and delicious brew, meticulously roasted to Steve's exacting standards.

I squeezed the Land Rover through the outsized stone gate jambs and down the drive between the coffee and banana plantations and the fenced sheep paddocks. Steve and loyal Katy Dog were in the yard to meet me, and after a quick look at Steve's pride and joy, a bronze Rolls Royce Silver Wraith, he led me through a set of latched gates via a walled vegetable garden and past a sprawling fig tree to the colossal duck pen. It was built against a high stone wall beneath Steve's beehives. Three more carcasses lay on the ground in poses of sudden death.

'It can't be the bees, can it?' Steve had once suffered several losses in his sheep when the flock had foraged between the hives and upset the volatile inhabitants. We had recently analysed their DNA, and they were essentially a St Helenian hybrid of the African killer bee. He and Maureen had put themselves at considerable risk to rescue their distraught animals.

'No, I don't think so. We'd see the stings around the eyes and there's no external swelling.'

'Poisoning?'

'Too sequential. It should be all at once. No, I think we have a genuine outbreak of some virulent disease. I'll take these dead ones and see if the findings are consistent.'

'After coffee, of course.' Steve, ever the gentleman, smiled affably and led me back to the warmth and fragrance of their traditional farmhouse kitchen. Pans bubbled on top of a Rayburn set deep into the old chimney breast as Maureen, a superb cook, prepared food for their guests.

'Come through to the veranda,' she said, carrying a tray with biscuits and dragging me along on a trail of coffee fumes.

Farm Lodge, a fully restored Georgian masterpiece bursting with antique furniture, lead crystal and silver plate, was Maureen's pride and joy and daily she toiled like a Trojan to abolish every speck of dirt and dust. The teak floors shone like water, everything was polished to gleaming newness. She would polish a pinhead. She would polish Steve (although salty seadogs take some polishing).

Beyond the veranda was Steve's domain, perfectly manicured lawns and an arboretum set in a vale of mature exotic trees gleaned from the trading routes of the East Indian Company. I savoured my coffee, basking in the period ambience, and resisting the temptation to strike the clapper of the bucket-sized ship's bell hanging from a beam that Steve had somehow rescued from the SS *Southern Cross*.

My next step was to research. The new post-mortems delivered exactly the same result, the pathology so precise that I knew it had to be pathognomonic – specific to one cause. I delved deep into the literature and before long struck gold in the US *National Parks Field Manual of Wildlife Diseases*. Microabscessation of the liver; pericarditis; myocardial haemorrhages; circling; flying upside down; even, alarmingly, falling out of the sky like an arcane, feathered bomb.

Fowl cholera.

This was serious. But before setting in train a whole cascade of legal actions, killing ducks and damaging livelihoods, I needed solid proof.

I moved on to the OIE – the World Organisation for Animal Health, now amusingly anglicised and re-acronymised to WOAH – and their terrestrial manual of diseases. Therein lay a handy tip. The causative agent is an anaerobic bacterium, *Pasteurella multocida*. The manual told me that this was a septicaemia and the bacterium should be found in profusion, but best of all, that it was subject to bipolar purple staining and should therefore be easy to detect.

I salvaged one of my semi-rigid post-mortems from an incineration sack and took a smear from the heart blood, stained it with dye and slipped it under the oil-immersion lens of the surgery's corroded microscope. And there they were, swarming between the duck's strangely oval, nucleated, red blood cells: legion upon legion of pretty purple dumbbell-shaped bacteria.

Now I knew my enemy, its strengths and its weaknesses. Time to formulate a battle plan.

LOCKDOWN

'Frank, I'm going to ruin your afternoon.'

Frank Wastell, the Attorney General, sized me up with a look of extreme tolerance. We were old friends and shared a similar brand of cynical humour. 'Well, that's a given considering you've just walked into my office.' Frank was a beneficial force on the island, a policeman who had pulled himself up by his bootstraps to become a lawyer. He worked tirelessly in the interests of the islanders, usually against the tide of bureaucracy.

'I need your help. We have a nasty disease outbreak which could spread over the whole island.'

'Look, I was perfectly happy until you walked in here bearing news of pestilence and Black Death, and now see what you've done. Curdled my tea. What disease?'

'Fowl cholera. In ducks. I have to quarantine Farm Lodge. Only I can't. The legislation says I must take it to committee and gazette it, and that's going to take for ever. Can you expedite it?'

'Ducks?' Frank exclaimed mockingly, then more seriously; 'Well yes, that's the Animal Diseases Ordinance for you, like most of our legislation positively antediluvian. How bad is it?'

I explained that internationally fowl cholera caused major die-offs in waterfowl, principally ducks, geese and swans, sometimes in their tens of thousands as the rotting carcasses contaminated the watercourses. But it could affect almost any species depending on the strain, so I couldn't rule out losing the endemic wirebird. Worse, the bacteria had a persistence of several weeks in the environment, Farm Lodge must now be hooching with them, and they could be carried and spread by rodents and wild birds around the island.

'Death and disease. Extinction. Avian Armageddon. Trust you. The voice of doom. Yes, leave it with me. I'll chase the chairman Lawson Henry and put the frighteners on him. He's a good chap and I'm sure he'll call an extraordinary meeting for tomorrow.'

Meanwhile, I went around to see Steve and Maureen and break the bad news.

'So,' said Steve, 'what does it mean?'

'Listen, I'm really, really sorry. But I'm going to have to euthanise all your ducks and place Farm Lodge under quarantine. That means no visitors except for those I issue a licence to, nothing to go off except under my authority, so no sales of eggs or vegetables. We'll place quarantine signs and disinfectant footbaths at the

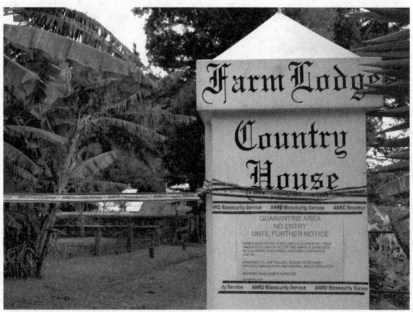

Farm Lodge goes into quarantine to prevent the spread of fowl cholera

entrance, and I have to tape off every gateway and footpath with our biosecurity tape.' To lock down somebody's business and forbid normal movement felt horribly autocratic.

'Hmm.' Steve pondered for a moment. 'How long for, do you reckon?'

'Probably a month. The actual duck pen, though, I would suggest, a lot longer. We'll work it out so we can get you back into business as soon as possible.'

'A month. Well, it has to be. We don't want this to spread either.' He sighed. 'Do what you have to do. As long as we don't have to wear bells around our necks and shout "UNCLEAN".'

'There's one other thing. The legislation has a defect. I can't declare quarantine until it's approved by committee and then gazetted. Can I ask you to observe these restrictions anyway? The local media have already got wind of it and are giving us a hard time.'

'Maureen?' checked Steve. She nodded. 'Yes, of course,' he said. It is rare to get such unreserved cooperation, but typical of Steve and Maureen.

THE INVISIBLE ENEMY

In 2001, rural UK slammed to a halt as foot-and-mouth disease burned through the country in an epidemic that has been esti-mated to have cost the public and private purse an eye-watering £8 billion.

For fifteen months in my home county of Devon I was immersed in the virus, treading the invisible line between clean and contaminated, having been called out to a suspect case in the Exmoor village of Clayhanger. It proved to be the last big county outbreak. I found my farm and all seven of its contig-uous premises (as they were so heartlessly labelled) absolutely saturated with the virus. It changed my work status from 'clean' vet to 'dirty' vet – since humans can carry the virus for up to two weeks in their tonsils – and my overalls from innocuous blue to stark white, used, almost perversely for all its clinical purity, to symbolise viral contamination. Backed by the army and police, we even chased the virus to linked premises across the Somerset border and stopped it in its tracks there. But only by slaughtering everything with cloven hooves. Even newborn lambs and lovely llamas. It was the worst of times.

That horrible experience did, though, mean that when it came to pathogen control, I knew my onions. I could never have predicted that it was to serve me so well on St Helena not once, but twice. This bout with fowl cholera, as it turned out, was only round one.

Full PPE with white suits over wash-down waterproofs; steel footbaths and buckets of disinfectant with jute hand brushes and six-inch nails bent into hoof picks for raking the mud out of the soles of our wellies; rolls of green and white sticky tape with 'ANRD Biosecurity Service' in thick, black letters to wrap around fence posts and stiles; and the mandatory laminated quarantine notices which I stuck to the gate jambs, marring their statuesque elegance with intimations of doom. The enemy was invisible, but it was everywhere, pouring out of the ducks, lying in wait to hitch a lift off the farm.

I briefed my small team, Ken and Andy, at the gateway. The fewer people on and off the premises the better. Andrea Timm, known to everyone as Andy, was my line manager, a sharply intelligent woman who was forever approachable and supportive. She was keen to be involved.

The three of us marched onto the farm, hooded and puffy in our spotless white suits, Ken and Andy carrying bags and tape, me a tray of kindly death: cotton wool and spirit, needles and syringes, and numerous bottles of pentobarbitone. Steve was waiting for us by the duck shed.

'The execution squad! For a moment there I thought my time had come.'

'How are things, Steve?'

'Forty dead, seventy to go, so this is for the best. They're all going to die anyway.'

Andy and Ken mustered the ducks and herded them into the shed while I charged several syringes with the violet barbiturate. Steve commented on its pleasant shade, and I explained that all the commercial euthanasia drugs were exotically dyed to warn the user what they were wielding in their hands. 'How nice,' he observed wryly, 'that death has a colour.'

One by one, we caught up the ducks, and while Steve and Andy restrained each bird, I plucked a pinch of feathers from under the wing, clarified the brachial vein with a swab, and injected a lethal dose of barbiturate. The third duck opted out.

'Andy, no point injecting this duck. You've a killer touch. It's dead already.'

'What? But I've only just caught it.'

Several others dropped dead in our hands. So it was true: they really do fall out of the sky, presumably from fatal heart attacks. Imagine that with geese. It would be a thoroughly unsettling experience to have one of those crashing through the foliage during a tranquil woodland walk.

Fortunately, Steve had the only large aggregation of waterfowl on the island. The bacteria failed to spread, the disease outbreak was contained, Frank amended the legislation to give the Senior Veterinary Officer seventy-two-hour emergency powers (council-lors don't like having their barbecues interrupted at weekends), and Farm Lodge was soon back in business. The status quo was thankfully restored – minus a few ducks.

Fate, however, has a warped sense of humour. All this was only a dress rehearsal for the real thing.

…INTO THE FIRE

Five months later, I was filling up with diesel at the fuel station in Half Tree Hollow, a sprawling suburb on the spartan hilltop just above Jamestown, when a woman approached me. She seemed distressed.

'Do you mind coming to check my chickens? I've lost three overnight. I live just round the corner.'

The woman had a dozen chickens in a wire-mesh pen below her house. I bagged the three corpses and noticed that one or two of the others had sagging wings and droopy combs. Some of the effluent from a nearby discharging pipe had seeped across the floor of the pen. 'Could be a poisoning,' I speculated. 'I'd get that fixed for a start.'

But the post-mortems were confusing. One had died of egg peritonitis, common enough in layers and similar in causation to an ectopic pregnancy. Another had a dramatic, mulberry-coloured trachea with grossly swollen comb and wattles. And the third had an ugly haemorrhagic enteritis and a weirdly gelatinous neck.

What the hell? I was baffled. A disease of many faces, every organ fair game.

A couple of days later I gave the woman a call to see how things were shaping up.

'Oh, the chickens are all dead,' she said, matter-of-factly. 'I've buried them.'

'Dead? All of them?'

'Yes, they all died soon after you saw them. I'll tell you another thing, though, if you're interested.'

'Please.' More than interested. Worried.

'Well, you know there are lots of wild chickens in Half Tree Hollow?' It was true; chickens everywhere, lurking in the scrub, rearing chicks on the cliff face, scavenging food from the rubbish sacks and the bins outside Solomon's bakery. 'They've all vanished.'

No, no, no, no, no. It wasn't possible. I was in denial. It had only been five months since the outbreak of fowl cholera, but this could only mean one thing: another disease, another pathogen with lethal capabilities. Only something far worse. This was a plague.

And slowly the pieces began to slot together. A pathogen that is fierce, that is merciless and swift, ransacking every organ, every tissue in the body within a short space of time, can kill in a hundred malevolent ways. It just depends which vital spark of metabolism is quenched first. My post-mortems varied because I was dealing with a highly virulent, highly fatal organism, a peracute infection attacking multiple systems simultaneously. Which might not exclude humans.

Last time, it was a bacterium. This time, given the ferocity, it had to be a virus. I had an inkling where this was going, and I didn't much like it.

Once again, I turned to the literature and, having more or less confirmed my suspicions, reached for the battered loose-leaf folder of handy notes, protocols and documents that I always carried around, a vade mecum accumulated over decades of practice. In it, I had stowed away a small bound booklet, issued by the Food and Agriculture Organisation (FAO), on handling birds with highly pathogenic avian influenza (HPAI), a disease of multiple viral strains. More commonly known as bird flu, HPAI occasionally infects and kills humans, mainly through close and intimate contact with infected fluids. It is a zoonosis, in fact. I had hoarded the manual with the far-fetched yet prescient notion that one day I might need it. That day had come.

The strains are named and distinguished by their H and N surface proteins. Avian influenza H7N9, for example, has a human case fatality rate of about 40 per cent, and H5N1 of about 50 per cent. Few cases but appalling odds. I was venturing into serious territory. Generally, these cases were chicken-to-human transmission, a dead end, but the great fear of epidemiologists is that one day the virus will mutate and launch human-to-human transmission: a pandemic. Something that the world is, by now, all too weary of.

But there is another virus that shares the symptoms of HPAI, causing a disease considered by some authorities such as the IUCN Species Survival Commission to be the most costly and socially

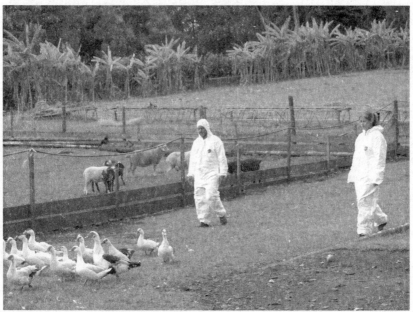

Mustering the doomed ducks for humane euthanasia

destructive of all veterinary diseases: Newcastle disease, named in 1927 after the first identified outbreak in Tyne and Wear, England.

Why is it socially destructive? Because chickens provide a staple, the egg, a rich source of vitamins, minerals, trace elements and high-quality protein, and they produce this marvel, an encapsulation of everything required to create a little chicky life, by recycling food scraps, organic waste, scrub and bugs.

Now, put aside the Western concept of popping into Waitrose and buying a slickly designed, Nile blue eggbox of a half-dozen free range eggs, and look at the reality facing the less fortunate, in their remote Ethiopian *tukuls*, Malaysian *kampongs* and Bolivian *pueblos*. Chickens control insect pests. They provide health-giving food. Crucially, they nourish the limbs of growing children. Next, picture a virus with a 100 per cent mortality rate sweeping through the land and destroying every single one of those chickens, and you'll quickly see the consequences, and how difficult, time-consuming and expensive it would be to replace the losses.

St Helena is not impoverished, but nor is it prosperous, and we'd worked hard through the importation of Lohmann Brown parent stock and our battery of government incubators to create a constant supply of fresh eggs to provide good nutrition and local income and to cut down on imports. Either way, whether Newcastle disease or avian influenza, we stood to lose everything. Possibly even human lives.

The similarity of the two diseases creates a confusion. On the one hand, you have a virus that could be the starting pistol for a pandemic and cost human lives; and on the other, a virus that is economically and socially devastating. Both important but for different reasons, and each with a different element of risk.

Unhappily, that confusion was now mine.

TWEEDLEDUM OR TWEEDLEDEE?

Fortunately, help was at hand. The OIE, FAO and EU had had the profound common sense to set up a chain of reference laboratories for this specific problem, and I was amazed and pleased to find them listed in the back of my prescient manual. The contact was one Professor Ian Brown of the Veterinary Laboratories Agency in Weybridge, Surrey. I phoned him.

'Yes,' he said, after I had told him my tale. 'Sounds like it's one of the two. Very interesting, though, because aren't you rather remote?'

'The second remotest island settlement after Tristan da Cunha,' I replied, repeating the oft-quoted mantra.

'For either of those diseases to reach you is a long stretch. Fascinating. And your isolation creates issues in getting the samples to us. We're going to have to freeze them, and that means creating a cold chain all the way to the lab here in the UK. But bear in mind these are live, infectious pathogens, so we need clearances.'

'I have an idea. The ship's coming in two weeks and then going to Ascension. I'll talk to our friends in the Royal Air Force.'

'Sounds good. But a warning. Neither the ship's captain nor the pilot has an obligation to carry the samples. You must get their permission. It's an internationally recognised courtesy. Meanwhile, I'll sort out the paperwork at this end and send you a sampling proto-col. And be careful. If it's avian influenza, you and your co-workers are at risk – especially when you're collecting the samples.'

'Understood. And if it's Newcastle?'

'At worst, snuffles and a touch of self-limiting conjunctivitis. But you may lose all your chickens and more besides. It's been found in almost 250 species of birds.'

It was Andy who brought the news. The virus had broken

out in a commercial flock belonging to her partner's father, Raymond, at New Ground, which was in direct line of sight of Half Tree Hollow. And it was, in the most ghoulish, spectacular way, shocking. I have never seen animals dying so fast.

Raymond's henhouse was a battleground. He had 130 laying hens, and the floor was littered with corpses. The living birds were barely living, fluffed up bundles lying on the ground in their final throes or standing forlornly with their wings hanging to the ground, their heads twisted over their backs and their combs an ugly purple. It would be a mercy to euthanise them.

Andy and Ken, fully trained by the fowl cholera outbreak and kitted up to the eyeballs, set to the task, while I toiled away at a makeshift table, dissecting the warm carcasses and collecting the requisite samples. I felt like a satanic butcher acquiring the essential ingredients for some vile, infernal feast: spleens, livers, kidneys, intestines, tracheas and lungs, with an *amuse-bouche* of cloacal and oral swabs. And fiddliest of all, brains; akin to wheedling out the soft, sticky centre from a very small, very hard-boiled and rather nasty sweet. That these samples had the potential to kill was a sobering thought.

Raymond was abjectly clearing away some of the debris. 'You know it's a funny thing,' he muttered, holding up a bleach-white egg. 'Lohmanns always lay brown eggs, but just the last day or so I've been getting these.' I smiled to myself and relaxed a little. A straw in the wind.

I had combed through reams of literature on avian influenza and Newcastle disease, and one paper – just one paper – had mentioned, in the long list of symptoms, that the shells of brown eggs tend to turn white with Newcastle disease, but are more commonly thin and rippled with avian influenza. I love the minutiae of diagnosis.

A second clue came later that day. I approached Senior Laboratory Technician Geoff Benjamin at the hospital for some robust outer sample containers, as the samples had to be triple sealed. In the absence of any veterinary laboratories on the island, Geoff had always been incredibly accommodating, and had even confirmed my fowl cholera diagnosis by enthusiastically growing the bacterium. 'I have something that might be of interest to you,' he said, proffering a small box. 'They're three years out of date but we've kept them fridged. A few years back, we were concerned about bird flu and brought in these nuclear protein bedside tests. You're welcome to use them.'

Ideal. I tested half a dozen samples and they were all negative. When I checked with Ian Brown, he approved. Not 100 per cent reliable, he said, but something to go on.

But the third clue was the clincher. I wouldn't normally be so elated to see a colleague of mine turned into a diagnostic tool, but Andy became the most excellent lab rat. She had sore eyes. Conjunctivitis.

'Andy,' I joked, grimly. 'Looks like we might live after all.'

It had to be Newcastle.

In any war, the key element in developing a strategy is to know your enemy, and ideally, to get ahead of its advance. I now knew my enemy and, with the RMS about to leave port in Cape Town, put in an emergency order for the best tactical weapon of all: vaccine.

THE SILVER BULLET

'It's the old morgue, but don't worry. No inmates!' Caz Yon, the European Space Agency's tracking station operator, was there to help as ever and showed me into the isolated building on Ascension's seafront, which stood a little distance from the main hospital. 'I'm sorry I couldn't be with you sooner but I had to track a rocket launch from French Guiana,' she added casually, as if she'd popped out to the corner shop to fetch a pint of milk. 'Altogether, then, we've got four dog castrations and three bitch spays.'

'It's perfect, Caz.' In the centre of the concrete floor was a long, self-draining, stainless-steel operating table, its true purpose only too clear. Outside, the equatorial sun beat down upon the lava-block walls, and turquoise waves lashed a sandy beach, but inside it was fittingly cool and peaceful.

The RMS had arrived at St Helena with the vaccines, and I had hopped aboard to courier the samples up to the RAF base on Ascension, now tightly packed, triple sealed and frozen in a huge cube of disinfected polystyrene smothered in officious labels. I leapfrogged the box from freezer to freezer and early that morning Caz and I drove out to the air base and handed it over. I had set the words 'ANIMAL PATHOGEN' in large, red font beneath the 'UN 3373' code and was amused to see how it provoked a raised eyebrow and a light, fingertip touch. The ship's captain and the RAF pilot were totally obliging. At RAF Brize Norton in Oxfordshire, a courier was to meet the plane and speed the box to the lab.

Meanwhile, I was performing my annual stint of duties for the quirky island of Ascension in its equally quirky capital, Georgetown. Amid its arcaded and gaily coloured military build-ings built of tufa, its coarse ash-cone forts, its black-mouthed naval guns gaping at the sea and its Victorian cast-iron ware-houses strung along the shoreline stands a delightful limewashed church with an amusing request pinned to its forest-green doors that unintentionally shuns – or maybe references – Jesus' mount for his ride into Jerusalem: 'ST MARY'S CHURCH •

WELCOME • PLEASE SHUT THE DOOR TO KEEP THE DONKEYS OUT'. Ascension is similar to, yet strikingly different from St Helena.

One of the striking differences is the existence of dazzling white beaches, entirely absent on St Helena. The main road through Georgetown drops down from the settlement into one of the most alluring of all, Long Beach, a curving half-mile of pristine sand beaten by Atlantic breakers, and here it is possible to witness a great spectacle. Every year, from January through to May, streams of green sea turtles migrate from the Brazilian coast to fight unfamiliar gravity and drag themselves up the beach at night, there to dig a crater in the safe zone, and lay and bury their eggs – over twenty-five thousand clutches a year.

Long Beach is so permanently cratered, it has the bombed-out appearance of Dunkirk. It wasn't hard to find a guiding caterpillar track made by a female in her colossal effort to reach higher beach. It led to her crater, where I found her scooping out sand with her powerful flippers, to then deposit a stream of lubricated ping-pong balls and cover them over. I watched this act of creation with that glow of wonder at nature's tenacity. The adaptation to those two great domains, land and sea, by two distinct but very similar chelonians, the giant tortoises under my care and the sea turtles under nature's care, is inspirational.

The very next day the results came through from the UK lab. Every sample, except for the brains, was positive by PCR for paramyxovirus-1: Newcastle disease. And thanks to the clues, we were already ahead of the epidemic. Back on St Helena the team were hard at it, vaccinating the nucleus flocks and ring-vaccinating New Ground and Half Tree Hollow, a first-line technique to wall off the spread.

Thanks to Frank's expeditious amending of our flawed ordinance, I'd had the power to quarantine each outbreak immediately and proceed with a cull. Nonetheless, I was convinced that the wild birds would hop the virus over the central ridge and infect the other side of the island, but the vaccine seemed to be stemming the tide. We had the public well on board with a 'Stop the Spread' campaign, so we decided to go the whole hog and vaccinate every chicken we could lay our hands on. To that end, we imported the LaSota vaccine, a highly practical live strain that could be given in the chickens' drinking water, but which had to be made up fresh and without any chlorination.

Andy organised a detailed delivery schedule and over the following weeks our Land Rovers parked up at strategic points like ice-cream vans, dispensing the vaccine diluted with rainwater in recycled plastic bottles. In this way, in their threes, fours, tens and twenties, we vaccinated over 5,000 chickens.

Proof of the vaccine's efficacy came in an unintended trial.

'I'm sorry, darlin'.' It was Gary Stevens, my favourite farmer, with his interesting West Country colloquialisms, surely introduced by roving Cornish sailors. 'I brought these ten in from Horse Ridge and mixed them in with the others, but they missed the vaccination.' Gary lived in Half Tree Hollow, now grossly contaminated with virus, and the ten new chickens were dying.

'Gary, you've just set up an interesting experiment. Normally I'd cull all the chickens, but I want to see what happens to the vaccinated group. I'm going to have to quarantine this area, but if I set you up with gloves and footbaths could you keep on feeding them?'

Gary loved a project. 'Oh yes, lurvie,' he replied gleefully.

Proof came: all the vaccinated chickens survived.

BOFFINS

After I'd attended to the animals on Ascension, I flew to RAF Brize Norton and drove down to the lab in Weybridge.

The lab is not one but many. It is a Biosafety Level 4 maximum containment laboratory complex and specialises not only in avian influenza and Newcastle disease, but classical swine fever, brucellosis, mad cow disease and the dreaded rabies. Ian and his colleague Ruth Manville were keen to show me around the maze of purposeful buildings, cunningly arrayed behind the brick facade of a former stately home. Around, of course, but not in, lest I wander off with some lethal microbe lodged in my hooves. Their enthusiasm was appropriately infectious.

We went to Ian's office. 'You have the worst form of the virus,' he said, with an undertone of supressed excitement. 'Viscerotropic velogenic, meaning it attacks the organs, it's fast and it's highly deadly. Mortality close to one hundred per cent.'

'Yes, that's what we're experiencing. I've never seen anything kill so effectively.'

'Well, I have to congratulate you,' he added. 'This is the remotest outbreak ever recorded, and I can only think that it reached you through imported poultry meat or eggs.'

'It makes sense.' I'd pondered on this long and hard. 'We don't have wheelie bins and the dogs and mynah birds rip open the rubbish bags looking for scraps.'

'Something else,' chipped in Ruth. There was a glint of the fanatical virologist in her eye. 'Look at this.'

She unrolled a large printout, a colourful family tree crammed with entries, and slid her index finger down the tightly bunched lines. 'All the reference labs share their data, and this is the family tree of Newcastle disease viruses going back decades, identified by certain key sequences in their RNA. They're all related. All except yours. The closest match is to a virus from central Africa way back in the 1990s, but frankly it's barely similar. The St Helena virus is unique.' Her finger came to rest on the last entry: St Helena, alone on the tip of its own, bare limb.

'How come?'

She shrugged. 'It's a mystery. Perhaps it came out of the jungle. But African countries sometimes fail to report their outbreaks. It may just be an unknown strain. What's interesting, though, is this isn't just a single mutation. There are lots of missing variants in between.'

'That is kind of fascinating.' I felt myself being sucked into their microscopic world.

'One other thing, Joe,' added Ian. 'It is of course a notifiable disease, and now we've officially confirmed it, you'll need to inform the OIE.'

'Yes, St Helena doesn't have a listing.' St Helena's frequent existential crisis. 'I'm on my way up to Nobel House in Westminster to sort it out.'

A few days later, when the listing came through, I informed the world. Not that the world particularly cared.

Over the several weeks of our vaccination campaign, we blocked the advance of the disease and killed off the epidemic. We had twelve separate outbreaks, with all cases confined to Half Tree Hollow and New Ground. Somehow the virus never made the leap over the central ridge; it perished, along with most of the feral chickens. Once again, vaccines saved the day – along with everybody's fried egg on toast.

There was just one enduring side-effect: never again could Andy stomach eating chicken.

There's still a tiny part of me, perhaps that tiny, fanatical virologist part they inoculated me with at the lab, that would like to cast a giant bronze of a Newcastle disease viral particle and place it in the Castle Gardens with the engraving 'KNOW YOUR ENEMY'. And underneath, in modest letters: 'Defeated 2014'.

It would confuse the hell out of the general public, but General Sun Tzu would surely have approved.

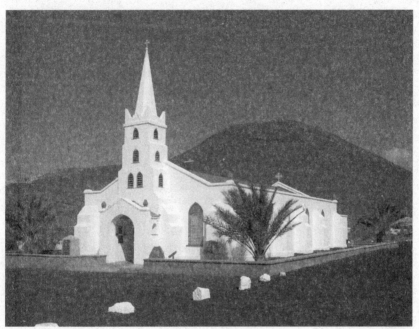

St Mary's Church, Georgetown, Ascension

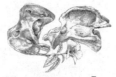

LEGACIES AND LEGENDS

The vessel contains ... little short of a thousand souls, which have been closely packed for many weeks together, in the hottest and most polluted of atmospheres. I went aboard ... as she cast anchor off Rupert's Valley ... and the whole deck ... was thickly strewn with ... dead, dying, and starved bodies.

John Charles Melliss, *ST. HELENA: A Physical, Historical,*
and Topographical Description of the Island, including
its Geology, Fauna, Flora, and Meteorology, 1875

POACHER TURNED GAMEKEEPER

'Is it human?'

Rob Kleinjan, Halcrow's environmental officer for the St Helena airport project, held out a grubby, angular bone, chipped and yellowed like ancient amber. He was cradling it in the palm of his hand with surprising tenderness, as if it were a fallen hatchling. His soft voice and lilting Dutch accent couldn't disguise his concern. 'We can't afford a delay like last time. They reckon there're up to eight thousand poor souls buried here.'

Eight thousand? Buried? We were standing by some excavations in the scoured floor of Rupert's Valley, surrounded by boulders, rubble and prickly pear.

There are only three places where the island's roads reach down to the Atlantic, so crumpled and tortuous is the landscape: Jamestown of course; Sandy Bay – on the opposite side of the island; and Rupert's Valley, the parallel ravine to Jamestown, almost a twin, though not as broad or as mighty. It was a fortunate whim of erosion that provided two bays, two anchorages and two settlement areas separated by a single ridge, Munden's Hill, so that the East India Company was able to seal both bays with curtain walls, connect the ravines with cliff-face bridle tracks complete with ringbolts for hauling cannon, and pile in numerous gun emplacements, some even pointing inland for rear assaults – or perhaps twitchy settlers. Unlike Jamestown, which is green, lush and abundant in its upper reaches thanks to the permanent gush of Chubb's Spring, Rupert's is a desolate valley. It could be the Badlands of Mexico.

As such, Rupert's was always destined to be the less loved servant settlement to Jamestown.

From the Boer POW desalination plant, the rare brick chimney now a national monument, to the more recent tuna canning factory, fish processing plant, bulk fuel tanks and island power station, Rupert's was always the place to tuck away the uglier, noisier and less comfortable aspects of St Helena's existence. And undoubtedly one of those less comfortable aspects, for the largest slave-trading nation in the world, was the African Liberation Depot, which was evidence of the poacher turned gamekeeper, dripping with guilt and hypocrisy.

Now here comes the history bit, but it's worth it.

For a tiny speck in the ocean, St Helena played a surprisingly significant and largely unacknowledged role in the abolition of slavery. The UK's Slavery Abolition Act of 1833 specifically excluded St Helena and so passed it by (though, it must be said, the East India Company, while once demanding a slave off every

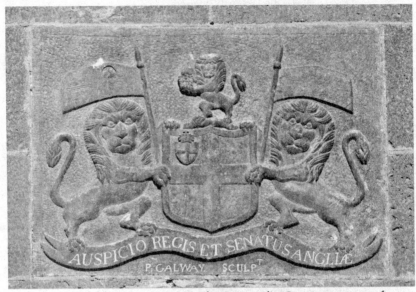

The East India Company coat of arms

ship en route from Madagascar in lieu of 'customs and dues', had made moves to unwind their role in slavery from 1774). By 1839 though, the abolition of slavery was technically achieved, although questionable 'apprenticeships' and other weaselly schemes stretched out its passing. Classical slave names such as Caesar, Scipio, Augustus, Hercules, Plato and Constantine persist as surnames on the island.

Then came the dramatic turnaround. If Britain ruled the waves, then, it was decided, it would also enforce its newly found ethics on the rest of the world. It would stop the abominable trade in Africans. Better late than never.

Much of the Americas had failed to follow suit. Britain decided that enough was enough, and evil participant became goody-two-shoes enforcer. With the earlier, much weaker legal prelude to abolition, the Slave Trade Act of 1807, the Admiralty in London had already established the West Africa Squadron, a small fleet of deft Royal Navy cruisers charged with intercepting and seizing slavers on the Middle Passage, the main slaving route from the west coast of Africa to the plantations of South America and the Caribbean. Now they could do so with greater zeal and alacrity.

But having seized a slaver vessel, what happens to the captives on it? It's not as if the average naval officer is likely to be fluent in the plethora of West African languages and dialects, and one pale-skinned European would be just as terrifying as another, especially when reinforced with roars of naval discipline, gleaming munitions and imposing uniforms all designed to cow a yielding vessel.

St Helena sat snugly and strategically near the Middle Passage. While many liberated Africans were returned to their coastal settlements, others who were of unknown origin or from subjugated tribes that had marched for weeks from the African interior were delivered to the African Liberation Depot in Rupert's Valley.

Between 1840 and 1864, 439 vessels were seized and delivered for adjudication to the specially established Vice-Admiralty Court in Jamestown, some empty but others packed in the most inhumane fashion with enslaved African people. Several Royal Navy cruisers were involved, with meaningful names such as HMS *Brisk*, *Wasp*, *Wizard*, *Fantome* and *Cyclops* – all implying unavoidable vigilance – but the most famous locally is HMS *Waterwitch*, originally an experimental racing yacht, so swift and nimble. She brought in forty-three slavers and a monument was later erected to her in the Castle Gardens.

In this way, 27,000 enslaved Africans were landed in Rupert's and theoretically liberated, ultimately adding to the Saints' genetic melting pot. Along with, I should add: indentured Chinese labourers brought in to build the roads, work the plantations and run a failed silk enterprise; officers of the East India Company and subsequently the Crown; lustful British planters with their feet firmly embedded in the island's soil; the odd Frenchman from Napoleon Bonaparte's extensive and expensive entourage; a few Boer prisoners of war who stayed; and lascars on shore leave doing what lascars on shore leave do. Throw in the Malaysian and Madagascan individuals who drifted in on the EIC's trading routes, and you have a genetically calorific recipe which makes the island population so wonderfully distinctive.

THE ABOMINABLE TRADE

In 2006, initial surveys began in Rupert's Valley for the prospective airport project. The airport site, the only terrain that had the potential for blasting out into a commercial airstrip, lay on the other side of the island on 300-metre cliffs at Prosperous Bay Plain. But to level ridges and fill gorges you need heavy machinery, for which you need a landing place and a connecting haulage road.

No ship had ever docked at St Helena; all movements of cargo and passengers had been carried out using motorised pontoons and lighters ferrying back and forth to ships moored offshore. Rupert's was to receive the first ever docking slipway, then a nine-mile-long haulage road was to be clawed out of the ravine to cross virgin hilltops and the hump of the island to finally reach the construction site. Only then could bulldozers and graders begin to flatten the landscape and join St Helena to the rest of the airborne world.

But then, in the path of all this planned construction, the surveyors stumbled across the grave of a formerly enslaved African. It turned out to be the first of many.

By 2008, osteo-archaeologist Andrew Pearson and his team had excavated an astonishing 325 skeletons to clear the way for the haulage road, but he estimated from surveys there would be some 8,000 in total, almost a third of the liberated Africans. For many, starved and subjected to unthinkable brutality, liberation had come too late. The renowned island chronicler of the times, John Melliss, summed it up when he boarded a captured slaver of near one thousand souls. 'Their limbs,' he recorded, 'were worn down to about the size of walking-sticks ... Many died as they passed from the ship to the boat.' The Trans-Atlantic Slave Trade database estimates that no fewer than 1.8 million Africans perished on the Middle Passage.

St Helena took its stewardship of the remains very seriously, and in 2020, after the completion of the airport project, the exhumed bones were reinterred in Rupert's Valley over a deeply moving weekend of remembrance, culminating in a ceremony of speeches, songs and reflections. The 325 wooden caskets were handcrafted by students from the local school, giving the younger generation a tangible connection with their past. The caskets were carefully stacked in a communal grave, each positioned as the bones had been found, lest mother be parted from child. Bouquets of arum lilies, which grow wild in the peaks, were laid on the lids, and the whole gently covered over. Chunks of magma, soaked in white emulsion, were set out on the flanking slope in giant numerals, a monument to the dead: '8 0 0 0', they cried.

I sang in our small choir, ably run by Teeny, a musician of rich ability, and I sang heartily, moved to tears. She had chosen a spiritual, 'Wade in the Water', reputed to have been used by the formerly enslaved abolitionist and activist Harriet Tubman to warn new escapees to flee into the river and conceal their scent from the slavers' dogs. A song, indeed, of liberation.

For me, it was also personal. I'm far from unique, of course, especially for many in the Americas, but some of my own forebears were survivors of the Middle Passage. Three per cent of my DNA – which shows a swirling mixture of Scandinavian, Germanic, Celtic and assorted Anglo-Saxon heritage – connects me to this abominable trade. One or more of my ancestors was ripped from the coastal region of Benin and Togo in exchange for manillas and trinkets, chained and manacled between stifling decks, and forced to lie prone, head to toe, with other captives, limbs enmeshed and fouled in excreta. It makes for hard reading, but don't look away. These are the depths of indifference to which the slavers sank, and we must never sweeten the depravity.

Clearly, he or she survived this unthinkable physical and emotional trauma, and I give thanks for it. Later, his or her descendant Margaret 'Ewers', a young enslaved African and my four-times great-grandmother, was manumitted and married, forcibly or otherwise, to Terence MacDermot, an Irish planter and owner of Holly Mount, an estate draped along the crest of the Jamaican Blue Mountains.

Evidence suggests she may have been gifted, in an obscene gesture of neighbourliness, by the adjacent Ewers plantation across the gorge. Margaret went on to bear MacDermot eight children. Whether this was a love match of some sort or a case of sexual subjugation, we can never know, but after three weeks researching in the archives at Spanish Town and a couple of days walking the estate up at Holly Mount, now devoted to growing coffee, I felt a kind of emotional connection to Margaret. So, forgive me, but in spite of the evidence and for peace of mind, I prefer to believe the former.

THE PIVOT

Rob watched me as I rotated the complex bone in both hands, contemplating its facets and articulations. 'Well? Do you think it's from a buried African? I really hope not.'

The haulage road had been completed, and the obliteration of Prosperous Bay Plain was in full swing, with thunderous detonations routinely shaking the core of the island. Every few weeks, a converted roll-on-roll-off estuary vessel going by the ungainly name of *NP Glory 4* hammered her way across the Atlantic from Walvis Bay in Namibia to press her blunt, equally ungainly nose against the new docking slipway and unload heavy machinery, ancillary equipment and tonnes of construction materials. The Atlantic is not an estuary, and by all accounts she sailed like a log. She had, nonetheless, made history as the first vessel ever to dock against the shores of St Helena. Now, the upper valley was being prepared for a row of bulk fuel storage tanks, and the excavations there had uncovered this bone.

'I'm not entirely sure. It's a cervical vertebra, a neck bone for sure. Leave it with me. I'll take good care of it and check it out.'

'As soon as you can, please. We've had to halt work.' Rob wasn't being insensitive; in fact he was never anything but pleasant, and very keen to be respectful of any human remains. But nevertheless, the works were on a schedule and he was tasked to deliver it.

The bone had endured many years beneath the soil of Rupert's but still retained its critical shape. There's much to marvel at in nature's designs, and the simple mechanical arrangement of the first and second cervical vertebrae is one such marvel. The first vertebra is called the atlas, rather neatly because like Atlas of Greek mythology supporting the globe of the earth, the atlas supports the globe of the head. It is more or less a hinge, allowing the skull to move up and down. The second is the axis, aptly named because it is the pivot around which the atlas can rotate. Put a hinge and a pivot in juxtaposition and you have a head that can bob and gyrate as well as any dashboard nodding dog. They are super-specialised and entirely different from the rest of the cervical vertebrae, and very distinctive between species. The bone I held had a protruding process, the odontoid peg. By sheer good luck it was an axis. Now all I had to do was match the species.

I thumbed through the dog-eared pages of my university anatomy book. Most veterinary books need regular updating, but anatomy books stay sound for a million years or so. The bone wasn't particularly large, and I soon dismissed cattle, sheep, goats and dogs, which just left horses. But surely it wasn't big enough? I turned to the chapter titled 'Equine Osteology' and, after cross-checking *Gray's Anatomy* to definitively rule out humans, I had my answer.

'Rob? It's Joe. I have some good news. You'll be relieved to hear you're not hacking through the grave of a poor liberated African. You've found the burial site of a small equid. In plain terms, a donkey.'

THE MONKAT IS BORN

I was soon back in Rupert's Valley, standing on the new slipway and attending to my duties with Pest Control and Biosecurity Officer Dr Jill Key, the doyenne of invasive species control throughout the Overseas Territories. Mundane though these duties were, especially in light of the burials in the valley floor beyond, they were about to generate a legend.

The one positive aspect of ships anchoring in the bay, especially on the leeward side of an island with a reliable offshore wind, was that any hitchhiking beasties, such as malarial mosquitos, venomous spiders or stowaway reptiles, had a challenge to make it ashore. Now that the inglorious NP *Glory 4* was butting her nose routinely against our shores, that safety net was gone. Worse in many ways, she was pouring cargo and containers onto the land on a regular basis. It was an impending danger.

In St Helena's benevolent climate, everything thrives: the beautiful, the ugly, the good and the very bad. While fruits and vegetables grow unhindered by frost, they are instead battered and brutalised by insect pests and diseases. The same applies to the island's fauna, though fortunately to a lesser extent, as they become infested by parasites introduced mainly from the interior of the African continent.

It wasn't always so. At the height of its strategic powers, the island could victual three ships a day, filling their holds with fruit and vegetables, and replenishing their barrels with water from the copious springs.

No longer. Worldwide, thanks to global warming and the increased movement of people, animals and produce, both legal and illegal, the biosecurity situation is getting worse. It's no longer a question of maintaining the status quo; the dam has already burst. St Helena imports most of its food.

Jill and I, along with the indomitable Julie Balchin, bio-security Rottweiler with the heart of a cream éclair, had the routine task of boarding the NP and clambering over the colossal pieces of construction machinery, peering into their cabs and chassis, checking puddles for mosquito larvae and probing every nook and cranny for lizards and newly spun webs. It was worth doing simply to be seen. The very first shipment delivered

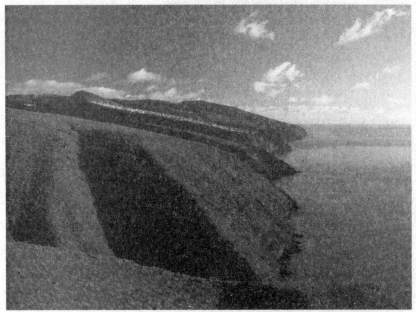

Towards Jamestown from Sugar Loaf

a telehandler with caterpillar tracks lagged in mud and chunks of vegetation, contrary to specified conditions in the contractor's 'design build and operate' contract. We gently reprimanded their operatives, banning its offloading until it was picked clean and all debris bagged and retained. Whereupon they ignored us and took it ashore.

We were outraged. The dirt was forgivable, a salutary lesson for all, but the behaviour was not. There is a massive void between a Namibian stevedore driving a machine through a muddy loading yard in Walvis Bay who has perhaps understandably given little thought to the significance of his action, and the managers at the top of the chain who squiggle their signatures on legal documents when they knowingly ought to be taking due precautions. It was our job to make sure the message reached up to supervisor level by correcting such issues pre-border. But this was treating us as a joke and flagrantly disobeying our orders.

And the telehandler was now illegally post-border – no better means of bringing ashore seeds, microbes, fungal spores and even nematode eggs. Thankfully, the threat of crippling fines from our no-nonsense head of customs, reinforced by our routine presence, soon meant that future shipments arrived factory clean.

Somehow, though, a biosecurity breach emanating from Rupert's seemed inevitable. But when it came, it wasn't at all in the form we could ever have predicted. It came in the form of a mythical beast. A chimera.

Nightwatchman Wavell Thomas protected the airport contractor's cargo area down by the foreshore in Rupert's. He was sitting in his chair in the early hours of the morning when he was approached by a strange, ugly creature with vertical ears, a flattish, hairy face and a long round tail. It was some thirty inches long and eighteen inches high – about the size of a springer spaniel – and brown in colour. The creature, he said, wasn't especially bothered by him and eventually sloped away.

Within days, Valerie Henry, who lived in a nearby stone mansion named Hay Town, also saw the beast standing on her garden wall. Then a second nightwatchman, Raymond Augustus, reported a similar sighting to Wavell's, giving an almost identical description and estimate of size, though he specified that it was a dirty grey colour. He had also heard an unusual animal scream during the night and observed that the prolific rabbits of the valley seemed to be holed up in their bunkers.

One sighting, a confusion or a waking dream. Three sightings in the same area and in quick succession, a reality. There was something prowling around in Rupert's. One description noted that, although catlike, the creature had the face of a monkey, and it wasn't long before one of the local papers, the *Sentinel*, coined a name: the Monkat. The police issued a statement, only reinforcing the beast's existence by advising the public not to approach any odd-looking, monkey-like creature, while the other paper, the *Independent*, went one further by commissioning an artist's impression, a chimeric half cat, half monkey with primate hands and sharp pointy ears. The Monkat was now firmly lodged in people's imaginations and gaining credence.

I was called down to Rupert's to examine some spoor – animal footprints – left in the mud. As soon as I received the call, I went online and expanded my knowledge on animal tracks by trawling through various hunting sites. I needed the woodsman's eye for detail, and pictured myself in the classic movie scene, perusing a single, smudged paw print and deducing that an aged lynx with a slight limp passed by five hours ago and paused to scratch a flea. The tracks were numerous and well impressed, and I didn't need second sight to say that they were the pawprints of a canid, though I was careful not to say a dog. I had picked up several key facts: that with the imprint of a canid's paw, which can include foxes, jackals and the like, you can draw an 'X' between the digital pads and the main stopper pad, but with the feline's paw print only a 'C'; that canids walk with fixed claws leaving an impression, whereas felines walk with retracted claws leaving no impression; that the canid print was oval, the feline's round; and that the stopper pad of a feline was a bubble 'M'. Nothing worse than a Google expert, but better than no expert at all.

The police called a gathering of various involved government entities, and the Chief of Police – yes, the COP – gave us a summary and his take on events. 'This,' he opined, 'is classic mass hysteria. The Monkat doesn't exist and we're not going to waste time hunting a myth.'

I had a different view. 'Myth or not,' I interjected, 'I have a professional duty to investigate the reports. I have no choice. Not to do so would be negligence, and it's not impossible that something has made it over here on the *NP Glory 4* or been dumped ashore by a yacht.'

I quoted the example of distant Tristan da Cunha where, bizarrely, some foolish yachtsman, presumably sick of having faeces hurled around the cabin, had dumped his pet monkey ashore at Sandy Point on the unoccupied east coast. It had had to be hunted down and shot. Nothing like a real-life example to tip the balance. Besides, I wasn't at all dismissive. In fact, I was intrigued, fascinated to see if the Monkat had flesh and bone. Jill Key heartily agreed, and we formulated a plan of action.

TRACKS, TRAPS AND THE DEVIL

Throughout history there have been regular sightings of exotic beasts in inappropriate places – the Beast of Bodmin Moor in Cornwall being one example from recent times – and because there have been genuine captures of large cats, released probably by panicking, impecunious or careless owners before and then because of the compulsory registration of wild animals, they are taken seriously. On St Helena we now had our own Beast, and the reports started to pour in. But so too, curiously, did myriad descriptions, and we were soon on the lookout for disparate incarnations of the same creature. The next sighting was at Chubb's Spring high in Jamestown Valley, just across the ridge from Rupert's. It was a fleeting glimpse, and the Monkat was described as cheetah-like, grey with dark stripes. Again, I was called to examine some spoor, both at Chubb's Spring and further up at the Heartshape Waterfall, a local beauty spot at the true head of Jamestown valley where a small stream casts a ribbon of water down a hundred-metre rock face. I had been told with some excitement that the prints were four inches long and had six pads, which seemed not only gargantuan but anatomically worrying. It turned out, however, to be a classic case of well-intentioned but overenthusiastic interpretation. I pointed out that canids and felines are zigzag walkers, placing their hind print neatly on top of their fore print. It was simply two overlaid impressions, hind on fore, and a canid's, probably a dog's. And certainly not a six-toed Cerberus straying from Hades.

The *Independent* put up a juicy reward of £300 for the first photograph of the Monkat, with the proviso that it was either captured or killed and clearly identified by the veterinary surgeon. That would be me then. The paper asked: 'Monkey, civet, jackal, caracal, mongoose or just a tomcat?', and published pictures of these suspects, further fuelling eager public speculation.

Jill, meanwhile, had laid out nine patches of soft sand at strategic locations in Rupert's, smoothed daily and ringed with movement-triggered camera traps, where she amassed a fine collection of dog, cat and rabbit prints, along with a few very human boot prints.

I quizzed the captain of the *NP* about whether it was at all possible that an animal could have sneaked aboard and made the six-day passage across the Atlantic unobserved. 'Absolutely not,' he told me, puffing up with indignation. 'I keep a spick-and-span vessel.'

Spick and span, yes, but I wasn't so sure. The *NP* was always loaded jam tight, and although I couldn't picture a wild feline skulking around unnoticed, I could imagine a canid, and six days spent licking up deck water was a feasible means of survival.

I knew that the docks at Walvis Bay on the Namibian coast stood alongside Flamingo Lagoon, a large saline wetland and wildlife sanctuary, with further wetlands just inland. Since the NP was a front-end-loader and docked with her ramp down, in my view there was ample scope for a hungry animal to sneak aboard at night. And if that animal happened to be pregnant, we'd soon have a pack of Monkats to contend with.

I even had a suspect in mind, equivalent to the urban fox: the black-backed jackal, a furtive scavenger that patrols the long coastal beaches of Namibia hunting birds and rodents and banqueting on rotting fish and seal carcasses. Its coat is brown and grey, and it has pointy ears and a round bushy tail. The only problem was the long canine snout.

I emailed the Namibian wildlife service. 'Sure', they confirmed, 'plenty of black-backed jackals around. And also,' they added, 'the wild cats hybridise with the domestic cats so they can be pretty big.'

Then came one of the most reliable sightings: two laboratory technicians at the hospital, Toni Joshua and Alexia Lawrence, both watched a dark brown, fox-like animal with a long, pointed face, pricked ears, and a thick fluffy tail stroll by at Maldivia, a luxuriant oasis area of upper Jamestown where mangos, avocados, pomegranates and bananas are grown. This came hot on the heels of another sighting by Shane Thomas in the Run, just below Maldivia. The Run is a linear park that brings the watercourse from the Heartshape Waterfall down through the heart of Jamestown in a handsomely masoned gulley. The path that runs alongside it is a shambolic mess, criss-crossing the gulley on planks and concrete slabs until the watercourse dives under the Iron Market and discharges into the sea, but the Run has great charm, giving insights into backyard Georgian Jamestown that are not to be seen from the street side of the buildings. Shane fumbled for his mobile phone, then froze. No photo and no reward; but his description almost exactly matched Toni and Alexia's. I became more convinced than ever that I was pursuing a jackal.

Time to think animal. I downloaded the cries of a pack of black-backed jackals onto a minidisc recorder and rigged it to the biggest speaker I could borrow. If there was a jackal out there, it would be confused, lost and lonely. I was going to woo it in its own language. All I needed was one reply, one telltale jackal howl, and I would prove its existence. In the evening light I drove up Jamestown Valley to the beginning of a disused carriage track, the Barnes Road, now a delightful, cliff-face hike that eventually surmounts the Heartshape Waterfall, and took up a lofty position on a crumbling stone wall overhanging the

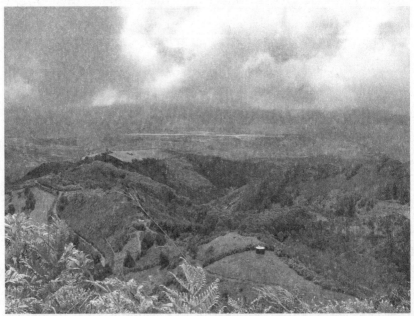

The newly constructed St Helena airport,
its runway visible on the horizon

deeply clefted valley. The valley floor at this point is uninhabited and densely vegetated, close to jungle. Since all the recent sightings had been heading in this direction, I calculated that from this vantage point I could fill the valley with enough sound to hook a homesick jackal.

I turned on the recorder and cranked up the volume. The woeful yelps and howls of the pack bounced and echoed off the soaring rock face opposite, reverberating from wall to wall until the whole valley seemed to resonate with legions of jackals. It was so effective that I almost felt intimidated. And so effective that, even though I drew a blank, I did manage to trigger a flurry of reports from tremulous upper Jamestown residents who had heard haunting, unearthly sounds emanating from the valley that night. There's nothing like stoking Monkat hysteria to new heights.

Our next plan was to try to trap the creature. Jill and I worked with hacksaw, wire and pliers to convert a dog cage into a scaled-up version of a rabbit trap, tweaking the homemade treadle and trigger rod for maximum sensitivity. We placed it in the Run and caught a cat. As the sightings gained momentum, she commissioned more traps from a local metal worker and scattered them around the key areas, catching more cats, a mynah bird and a miscreant dog.

Strange noises were heard in Plantation Forest, the eerily beautiful mature woodland of fat-limbed cape yews and clattering thickets of giant bamboo that lies in a small vale alongside the Governor's palatial residence. When beckoned by the representative of the Crown one must respond, and a trap was duly set.

A couple of days later, Jill collared me at work. Something had tickled her mischievous sense of humour. 'The trap in

Plantation...' she began. 'It was triggered and the bait was gone, but we didn't catch anything. We did, though, have some footprints around the trap.'

'Oh,' I replied, genuinely interested as I now considered myself the local tracking expert. 'What sort?'

'Cloven hooves!'

There are no sheep, goats, cattle or pigs anywhere near Plantation Forest. 'Are you telling me...?'

'Yes,' she cut in, barely containing her amusement. 'It does appear that the Monkat is from another realm. The Devil is stalking the forest.'

The Saints are fairly superstitious on the whole: you can often hear talk of mass hauntings, the Evil Eye and the Gilly Gilly. I had myself once been placed under the spell of the Gilly Gilly, my Saint colleagues told me, after emphatically advising a goat owner to slaughter her kid goat with a fractured femur because it certainly wasn't worth fixing. She smiled warmly, interlocked her fingers and rotated her thumbs to cast the spell; and I promptly changed my mind. I took the kid goat back to the clinic and performed what in the UK would have been a thousand-pound orthopaedic operation for a tenner. She did, though, give me some bananas. The Gilly Gilly is a trick I've since tried to master but with disappointingly limited results.

We decided therefore that, however funny the thought was, it was probably best not to publicise our finding of cloven hooves in Plantation Forest. Unimaginative though it may be, I drew the line at the Devil playing pranks on us – I preferred the rather dull explanation that someone's ram had probably gone wandering, looking for a lucky chance.

Then one of my talented team, Rico Williams, blew apart my firmly held belief of a black-backed jackal. 'Hey, Joe, sorry to spoil your theory, but you know those clear sightings in the Run and up at the hospital? That's Stewie's dog, Ellie. She must have got out. Stewie lives just above in Maldivia.'

Stewie's dog was a Belgian Malinois and a convincing stand-in for a small wolf or jackal. She was also a trained attack dog used for drug detection and security patrols and had the air of a wild animal about her. Shane had been right to freeze in the Run; it was probably instinctive.

The sightings began to multiply. At Kunji Field, just alongside Plantation Forest, an expat glimpsed a strange animal diving through the hedgerow in his car headlights, but it was late at night and the description was vague. In Clay Gut half a mile away there were several reports, but the descriptions were increasingly contradictory: short legs, stout legs; small ears, round ears, triangular ears; lioness tail, long tail, straight tail with black rings; black and grey body, beige body, speckled body, white underbelly, and most intriguing of all, curry powder mixed with soot and a dirty white rear. I had no doubt that all these reports were given in good faith and an animal was being seen; just not necessarily the same one each time. Circumstantial observations were reported in the newspapers: someone heard an animal walk across his roof at night and found the rubbish bag torn open in the morning; all the dogs barked at once; strange caterwauling was heard; a mauled rabbit carcass was found. Nothing substantial, in fact nothing out of the ordinary at all. But imaginations were heightened all over the island.

ABSENCE OF EVIDENCE IS NOT EVIDENCE OF ABSENCE
It took three months for the sightings to abate. Although part of me was disappointed not to come jowl to whisker with the Monkat, another part of me – the rebellious streak – was glad.

It would have been my sad professional duty to kill it, to debunk and destroy a myth. Instead, it may have roamed off into the wilder tracts of the island, feasting on the bounty of rats and rabbits, and acclimatising to a new, unexpected habitat across the Atlantic. A permanent holiday perhaps.

Did the creature exist? I like to think so. There was definitely some animal of unusual appearance prowling around Rupert's. It could have been dumped by a yacht, it could have sneaked off the *NP Glory 4*, or perhaps more realistically, it might have been a huge and hungry old feral tomcat, drawn in from the wilderness by the aroma of cooking or Wavell's liver pâté sandwiches. I even had a theory that the reported ugliness of the creature's face could be explained by the ravages of cancer. The island's cats have a tragic susceptibility to sun-induced malignancies of unpigmented noses, ears and eyes caused by the high levels of ultraviolet radiation, and it's in a cat's disposition to ignore veterinary advice and sunbathe. I have performed many ear amputations and eye enucleations, and on several occasions, euthanasia when a carcinoma of the nose has eaten away the middle of a cat's face, giving it a cruelly monstrous appearance.

Perhaps one day someone clearing a densely foliaged gut will come across the bones of an alien creature and put the mystery to rest. But I hope not. I like a mystery. It is a scientific axiom that it is easier to prove the existence of something than the non-existence of something. There is no possible evidence that can disprove the Monkat's existence, and it will always possess an otherworldly mystery that feeds and stirs the imaginations of the islanders. And there's no harm in that.

The other day, hanging in a shop window, I was brought up short by the sight of a brightly coloured, souvenir tea towel designed for tourists. It depicted key features, beauty spots and historic sites, all illustrated within a sea-washed outline of the island. In the centre was an outlandish creature with a monkey's face, and underneath the words: 'The Monkat'.

The Monkat is now firmly embedded in island folklore.

The Monkat lives on.

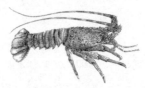

At the End of the Earth

We, the undersigned, having entered into co-partnership on the island of Tristan da Cunha, have voluntarily entered into the following agreement. Viz:

1st – That the stock and stores of every description in possession of the Firm shall be considered as belonging equally to each ~

2nd – That whatever profit may arise from the concern shall be equally divided ~

3rd – The purchases to be paid for equally by each ~

4th – That in order to ensure the harmony of the Firm, no member shall assume any superiority whatever, but all to be considered equal in every respect, each performing his proportion of labour, if not prevented by sickness...

Signed: Samuel Burnell, William Glass, John Nankivel

Agreement on the establishment of the colony,
Somerset Camp, Tristan da Cunha, 7 November 1817

A GLASS LINK

There was an island I had always wanted to visit, but I knew I never would: Tristan da Cunha, the remotest island settlement in the world.

Tristan was 1,500 miles away and simply too inaccessible. Even the St Helenian governors – a role which encompassed governorship of Tristan – generally had trouble visiting and some never managed it during their term of office. Since the RMS had cut Tristan out of her route, and with her rapidly approaching replacement by the new airport that was still being ground out of the igneous chaos on Prosperous Bay Plain, the only way of getting there was by fishing boat, returning once the holds were packed with frozen crayfish. Somewhat too rough and leisurely for the Crown's representative.

But one evening, I was invited by Sean Burns, Deputy Governor of St Helena and one-time Administrator for Tristan (and soon to be again), to a welcoming party at the Briars Pavilion for two visiting Tristanians, Julian Repetto and Trevor Glass, up from the island on an information exchange. Trevor's ancestor, Corporal William Glass, was the founder of the island settlement.

The Pavilion is a French domain, Napoleon's first, brief house of exile and his only happy one. It is exquisitely maintained by the Honorary French Consul, Michel Dancoisne-Martineau, a man of immaculate taste. It is a stunning venue, an architecturally imaginative and beautifully decorated building dripping with antiquities. I stood on the raised veranda, washing a smoked salmon canapé down with a luscious red wine, assuaging my frustrated curiosity by chatting to Trevor about Tristan, where he headed Conservation. He was relaxed and friendly, with a delightful musical accent and a wicked sense of humour. We bonded with no difficulty at all, and he asked to shadow my work during his time on St Helena so that he could get to know our island and garner a few extra skills to take back to Tristan.

A few weeks later, we were up at the sheep pound at Man & Horse, a onetime lookout. The sheep syndicates of Man & Horse and Botleys Ley are designed to share out limited pasture to groups of islanders, and are confined to the Western Pastures, rolling hills set atop titanic sea cliffs of breathtaking beauty that taper off into the south-western tip of the island. The pounds are a gathering of the sheep for routine husbandry and my favourite of all the island's social occasions. The syndicate members banter and guffaw with rich, merciless, rustic humour as they drench, shear, tag and castrate. Chief among them, Gary Stevens.

Gary had an artistic skill; he could whittle ears. With the tiny, scalpel-sharp blade of his pocket penknife engulfed in the ham of his hand, he excised small symbols from the left and right ears of the newborn lambs with the refined dexterity of a plastic surgeon: swallow tails, fleur-de-lys, crops, slits and notches. Within syndicates, this slight mutilation, unpleasant but necessary, establishes a permanent mark of ownership.

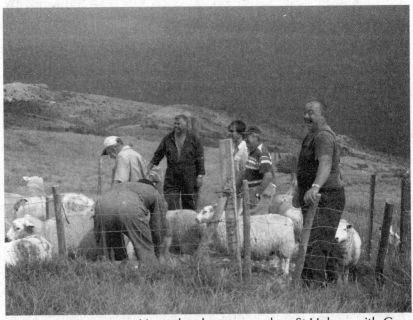

Up at the sheep pound on St Helena with Gary
Stevens, Trevor Glass and others

Although plastic ear tags are also used, they fail. There seems to be no design in the world that can survive the rough grazing and strong ultraviolet light of St Helena. Ear marking is the failsafe back-up.

Trevor participated to the full. He could have been Gary's long-lost brother, similar Buddha build, similar warm wit, similar charismatic charm. Belly laughs abounded. The pound was hot, hard work, as every sheep was pushed through the race, drenched and checked, every lamb examined, docked and ear marked, and if a male, castrated with an elastrator. After, we lay out on the turf in our lofty field, mighty oceanic views all around, drinking tea and having a bite to eat.

Which is when Trevor rolled onto his side, turned towards me with a conspiratorial grin and said: 'I've booked you on a ship to Tristan.'

SLOW BOAT TO GO REMOTE

The MV *Baltic Trader* sailed like a dustbin. Badly.

We were several days out from Cape Town on a 1,700-mile voyage to Tristan da Cunha, an island of some 250 souls, and it wasn't going too brilliantly.

The *Baltic Trader* was old, blunt nosed, and round bellied with a shallow draught. The winds were head on, the seas mountainous, and with every dive into the deep troughs she would headbutt the face of the oncoming wave, judder to a near halt, pitch, roll and corkscrew as she wallowed from the blow, then slowly claw back some headway. Like a punch-drunk boxer who just won't go down. Fortunately.

A voyage of some seven days, we had been told, but the software on the Polish captain's laptop was now estimating an alarming eighteen to twenty-one days. We were going to the remotest island settlement in the world on the slowest ship in the world.

'It's a disaster,' he said. He was a charming, educated man who allowed us to wander the bridge at will. 'But what can you do?' The bosun, a dark-skinned Cuban with gold-capped teeth, smiled expensively in agreement. The majority of the crew were Ukrainian. 'It should, though, improve once the wind comes from behind.' We all love an eternal optimist.

Tristan da Cunha has a remarkable resource: crayfish. *Jasus tristani.* So many crayfish that they wander the kelp forests like an infestation of ants, can be picked out of rockpools at low tide, and even used to clamber up the hemp cables of ships anchored offshore. Between the four islands of the Tristan da Cunha archipelago – Nightingale, Inaccessible, Gough and Tristan – some 400 tonnes are harvested annually, the backbone of the island's economy. It is a carefully assessed resource and is fished to quota.

The fishery is managed by Ovenstone, which by agreement also uses its vessels for cargo supplies and up to twelve passengers at a time, including medevacs. So here we were, a motley bunch, on our way to Tristan: GP Dr Martin; audiologist Dr Jane and her husband Ian; Clint the crayfish factory manager and his wife, permanently confined to cabin by seasickness; Paul, Geri and their two young daughters, and Nicky – my first Tristanians. Not to forget three lovely pups: a bouncy pair of collies and a cheeky little fluffball of a Maltese terrier.

By day three, we were a plague ship. Geri and her daughters were covered in the itchy scabs of chickenpox, and there was a chance Tristan would refuse us landing. Paul and Nicky were on puppy-poo patrol, and all the pups developed diarrhoea; in their characteristic puppyish way, they kept bouncing up and down and plastering them both with liquid faeces. Whereupon Paul and Nicky would saunter back into our midst reeking like a cesspit.

The days passed with predictable monotony: food, games of Scrabble, stare at the wake, more food, more games of Scrabble, stare at the wake. No internet, no contact with the outside world. Just the constant throb of the engine, the shuddering hull, and a shipless ocean with an encircling army of cresting waves. The Capetonian chef spoiled us with vats of thick stew and exquisite bread-and-butter puddings. The captain made his signature dish, a coronary cake of caramelised condensed milk, cream and chocolate, still promising us that the vessel's speed would pick up. Which, mercifully, eventually, it did.

By day eight, while I was standing on the wing of the bridge with Dr Jane, a wandering albatross glided alongside, slipstreaming the ship so closely that we marvelled to hear the wind ruffling the feathers along its remarkable ten-foot wingspan. When the shearwaters began to follow in our wake, we knew land was somewhere over the horizon.

By day ten we were finally approaching the island, but the weather had deteriorated, and rain was pelting the portholes and flowing across the deck in rivulets. Even at three miles distant, the massive 2,000-metre conical volcano that forms the island was totally concealed, and yet there it undeniably was, blipping on the radar. The wind had swung into the worst direction, north-west, straight into the mouth of the tight and fickle harbour entrance, and we were shaving the day; the light was failing rapidly.

We were keen to land but knew that sometimes it could take a week for the weather to settle sufficiently to take off passengers and cargo. We joked half-heartedly about the Voyage of the Damned while Nicky and the coxswain of the motorised pontoon debated the feasibility of disembarkation on the radio. At least the chickenpox had run its course and Geri had finally been able to shampoo the cornflakes from her scalp.

A menacing, black cliff of jagged, tumbled magma, a remnant of the 1961 surprise eruption, suddenly materialised out of the murk.

'Look, look.' I was pointing, barely able to contain my excitement. In the crepuscular light, we could see the ghostly glimmer of scattered houses on a sloping settlement plain, and an imposing 800-metre escarpment towering behind.

At last.

Edinburgh of the Seven Seas, known locally as the Village or the Settlement.

It was decided. A landing was to be attempted. We stacked our luggage on the hatch of the forward hold, where it steeped in the cold, pelleting rain, and a motorised pontoon materialised from the intensifying dark. A small team of Tristanians in glossy black oilskins swarmed up a rope ladder and busied themselves with our evacuation onto land. The ship's derrick swung our small passenger cage off the deck onto the pitching pontoon and we quickly fled for the safety of the harbour.

Calshot Harbour is fabricated from two outstretched arms of dolosse – giant, geometric, interlocking, concrete knuckle bones – since Tristan's natural harbour at Big Beach was buried for ever under magma. The entrance is narrow, and the storm was hurling breakers straight down its throat. In the now stark, black night and driving rain, the coxswain charged the gap at full power, caught a wave crest and surfed the pontoon into the relative tranquillity of the harbour. A dramatic arrival. Extreme remoteness should never be easy to reach or it's not remote.

All my life I have been around the sea, and I could immediately recognise hardy, accomplished seafolk. My instinct was soon proved right. I would see how Tristanians live by the sea, with it, on it, from it. They respect its power, cherish its gifts and abide by its rules. They are highly attuned to its mercurial temperament and can read its moods and converse in its language. And when it knocks them down, they get right back up again.

A large reception crowd had gathered on the stone wharf, shining in waterproofs under the quayside lights. The Administrator, the recently returned Sean Burns, water dripping from his hood, welcomed us with a handshake. An older man with a gruff Scottish accent sought me out and introduced himself: Alasdair Wylie, the agronomist, soon to become my comrade-in-arms. And then Iris and Martin Green, my hosts for the next two weeks until I settled into more permanent accommodation, who led me to their house on the edge of the Village and looked after me royally with sufficient food for a pod of whales.

Ahead of me lay nearly a year of intense experiences. Tristan da Cunha was to get into my blood, into my very bone marrow, in a way I could never have predicted. But my time there was to have an ugly start. What I didn't know then, what none of us knew, was that we were on the brink of a meteorological catastrophe.

UTOPIA

Why on earth is there a British Overseas Territory in such an apparently futile location? We only have time here for a potted history, but it boils down to one name: Napoleon.

Tristan was discovered in 1506 by the Portuguese admiral Tristão d'Acunha, hence the name – somewhat garbled down the years – but the first true settler was an American, some say a privateer, called Jonathon Lambert. He changed the name of the archipelago to the Islands of Refreshment and his camp to Reception, in a bid to lure ships in for trade, but swiftly drowned in a suspicious boating accident, leaving behind one poor wretch to tell the tale. Rumours of Lambert's buried treasure linger even today – though the cache was probably just potatoes.

In 1815, after Napoleon finally succumbed at the Battle of Waterloo, he was sent to St Helena, his second place of exile after his resurgence from the Isle of Elba. Elba had been a gentlemanly compromise, flanked as it is by Italy, France and homely Corsica. But Boney hadn't 'played cricket'. Second time around, the usual courtesies were thrown to the dogs, and the British cast him out into the remote fastnesses of the mid-Atlantic. But, now suitably paranoid, they also established a garrison on Tristan da Cunha, claiming the island in 1816 on behalf of King George III to prevent a French backdoor operation springing Napoleon from captivity.

When the pointlessness of this garrison – some 1,500 miles from Napoleon's captivity on St Helena – eventually became apparent, it was withdrawn, but a Scottish corporal, William Glass, appealed to stay and continue to fly the flag for Britain, along with his wife, children, and two Devonian stonemasons. His request was granted, and the settlement was born.

The three men then drew up a co-partnership agreement which formed the basis of a mini-utopia: that stocks and stores belonged equally, that all profit be equally divided, that purchases be paid for equally, and that all members be considered equal in every respect and not assume any superiority. Although this was amended in 1821 to take account of an expanding population, it has undoubtedly instilled a lasting and profoundly impressive character of mutuality, self-reliance and community spirit that was soon to sweep me up and embrace me.

The population waxed and waned. By 1826, there were William Glass and his family, and five frustrated bachelors, but Captain Simon Amm of the ship *Duke of Gloucester* made an appeal to the ladies of St Helena and brought back five new consorts for the single men – allegedly in exchange for a sack of potatoes each. Cold nights being what they are, the numbers boomed. In 1885, the most horrific of events nearly destroyed the settlement when fifteen of the island's men were lost at sea while attempting to trade with a passing vessel. They left behind thirteen widows and a devastated community.

But the Tristanians are never ones to give up. A succession of shipwrecks and passing whalers added to the community. Key among them was the sinking of the barque *Italia* out of Camogli in Italy, bringing two new family names to the island, Repetto and Lavarello, along with the Mediterranean design of the Tristanian longboat, which would play a crucial part in the islanders' bonding with the sea and its neighbouring islands.

The net result, including subsequent settlers, is just seven principal family names: Green, Hagan, Swain, Rogers, Repetto, Lavarello and of course Glass. As I came to know the Tristanians, I could see in their various features the Afro-Asian influence of the Saints, the fair complexion of the Scots, and the olive colouring of the Italians: a beautifully diverse mix of origins.

EDINBURGH OF THE SEVEN SEAS

I woke to the sounds of a church bell and a burbling stream. The storm had abated. It was Sunday morning and time to explore the Settlement.

Picture a small tangle of concrete tracks on a grassy slope and, arranged among the looping tracks, neat, single-storey cottages with tin and corrugated asbestos roofs, huddled comfortably in pairs, threes and fours, some with bulging gables of cocoa stone – volcanic tufa that has been hewn with a hand axe into different-sized blocks then jigsawed together as seamlessly as the Inca masonry of Machu Picchu.

Around the cottages, tall stands of New Zealand flax, once used for thatching and now as effective windbreaks, mesh with colourful slatted fences and latched garden gates to enclose treasured little gardens. Immediately above the harbour stands the modern crayfish factory – a third incarnation after the second burned down – a collection of warehouses, a single supermarket and the government offices. And in a central loop sits the hub of social events: the Prince Philip Hall with its indispensable Albatross Bar. Add to this the occasional herd of beef suckler cows wandering through trailing thirsty calves, plus numerous dogs – principally working collies – ducks with trains of ducklings, and assorted multi-coloured chickens, and you begin to see the Settlement. Don't include cats; there are none.

Now surround this fine, bucolic scene with a pair of gullies running out to sea and pastures seamed with black volcanic walls, and seal the backdrop with the impassive, green-grey face of the 800-metre escarpment.

The gullies differ significantly. To the west a deep, ragged scar called Hottentot Gulch – an Afrikaans name coined long before the transit of time showed it up as racially insensitive – crossed by a track heading out across the Settlement Plain to the Potato Patches. To the east, the Big Watron – 'water run' – an endless gush of pure, crystal mineral water that bursts from the foot of the escarpment into beds of watercress and tumbles down through the pasture in a boulder-strewn stream, running right past my accommodation. It supplies the Village and, once upon a time, filled the barrels of passing ships with copious, delectably sweet water.

There's one other feature we must add to the picture, because it is so significant, so historically important. The crouching black monster of the 1961 volcano.

I had always imagined that the Tristan eruption had been from the main crater 2,000 metres above sea level. Not at all. It was from a leak just 100 metres above.

The Settlement Plain was formed by erosion taking a chunk out of the north-west side of the conical island, like a bite from an apple. But this erosion created a weakness in the cap over the roiling magma chamber in the bowels of the volcano below. In 1961, the magma chamber became agitated, the magma rose, huge cracks opened and closed, trapping and swallowing sheep, and a spew hole burst forth within metres of the Settlement. Rivers of molten rock oozed down to the sea, flattening the first crayfish factory and filling in Big Beach where the longboats were pulled up, building into a cruel, black, craggy arm with crusty, knuckled cliffs. It severed the eastern end of the Settlement Plain, leaving a remnant pasture with the evocative name of Pig Bite.

The islanders were evacuated to Nightingale Island and then on to the UK. It must be so tragic and disheartening to leave your way of life, your home, your island nation for ever because it has been irrevocably destroyed. To abandon your dogs, sheep and cattle to an unknown fate, and to face yourself an uncertain future.

And yet... and yet... Quite remarkably, as various survey ships were sent to monitor the situation, it was discovered that the Settlement had been spared. In 1963 the Tristanians returned. I had occasion to talk to a fine old gentleman and ex-Chief Islander, eighty-three-year-old Harold Green, while taking tea and cake in his comfortable parlour, and he recounted the evacuation. He spoke movingly of the survival of the Settlement in his soft, warmly accented voice.

'If the lava turned left and come this way, there'd be nothing left, but it turned right, clean round the Little Beach, and God put his arm around the Settlement and said, "Look. You're safe."'

No greater reminder can there be, no greater monument to the reprieve of the Village, than the louring mini-volcano and its frozen rivers of magma, now designated as a public park.

BEFORE THE DELUGE

Monday, my first day of work, and I sat in the Head of Agriculture Neil Swain's office going through old reports. The door opened, and a tall, handsome man with bright, intelligent eyes and a broad, white smile leaned in, holding out my freshly stamped passport. He was immaculately dressed from head to toe in British police uniform.

'There you are,' he said. 'You're all official, stamped in to the island for the foreseeable future.' The stamp depicted a conical volcano overlaid by a spread-winged albatross. 'Lewis Glass,' he added, by way of introduction. 'Filling in for Connie Glass while he's away.'

Lewis was to become my landlord when I made my move to permanent accommodation, and was a man whose wit, wisdom and company I could never get enough of. His long, stone-gabled cottage stood at the very top of the Settlement, a cinder's throw from the 1961 volcano, tucked in the corner of the rear lava wall that separated all the cottages from the pasture called Back Fence. It was right on the bank of the gushing Big Watron, which burbled me to sleep nightly. 'Fence', I soon came to understand, meant 'field' in the local parlance, and Back Fence acted as a shield against the regular rockfalls from the dominating escarpment to which cattle often fell victim. It was a homely arrangement: he lived in one end of the cottage with his wife Yvonne, and I lived in the other end. It was the only cottage to be damaged during the 1961 eruption, when the thatch was ignited by some fiery debris. I revelled in its congeniality, its history, its outlook and the warm hospitality of Lewis and Yvonne.

Neil showed me to my office, a rusty dark-blue shipping container which I shared with Alasdair, and which flooded every time it rained. Yet I liked its bright airy atmosphere and the company of the wise old agronomist. He also introduced me to Dereck Rogers, the veterinary officer and my Tristanian counterpart, short and stout, immensely friendly, and crammed with invaluable local knowledge, which I tapped into keenly.

Neil struggled with a voice complaint and had even been to Harley Street in London for treatment, but he always fought valiantly to make himself understood, and it was clear to me I was in good hands. 'This is Ray Green the herdsman,' Neil croaked, indicating a slim, chirpy figure with a balding head and the universal welcoming smile. 'He's going to take you on a tour of the Settlement Plain so you can get the lie of the land.'

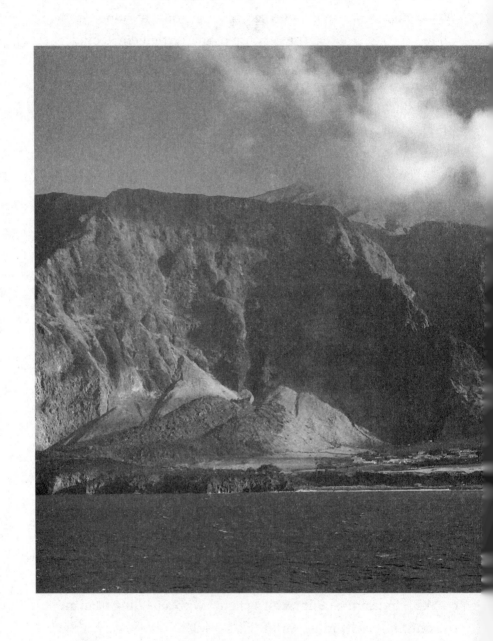

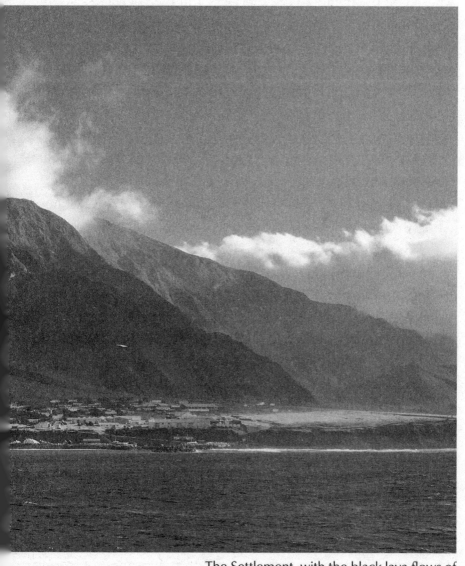

The Settlement, with the black lava flows of
the 1961 eruption visible to the left

We jump-started a clapped-out Toyota, Agriculture's flogged workhorse, and rattled up through the Settlement with Ray acting as tour guide, funny and relentlessly enthusiastic as he reeled off the names of the paddocks and their acreages.

In the heart of the Settlement: American Fence, which was grazed by the Village herd and cradled the graveyards, walled clusters of white headstones including that of Corporal William Glass, the founder. Then Easter Fence, wedged between the Big Watron, the 1961 volcano and my backyard. We pottered along the top of the Settlement, parallel to Back Fence, and down into Ginny's Watron, grounding the exhaust in the dip.

A succession of pasture names trickled from Ray's lips: Bugsy Hole, Valley, Spring Fence, Calf Piece, Long Piece, Top and Bottom Wash, Shateller's Hut, Top and Bottom Mudhole, and lastly Burnt Wood and The Bluff. There an oblique cliff cuts off the final piece of steep pasture, Anchor Stock, from where, one day, I watched entranced as Tristanians brought the ewes back for lambing by driving them in long, white threads along unseeable, cliff-face toeholds.

But the highlight was an amble around the Potato Patches, lovely chequerboards of small, square enclosures, walled with rough chunks of frothed, black lava to keep out the cattle and break the scourging effect of the salt-laden gales.

The common spud. My Irish blood cherished the Tristanian potato, a staple food for the Tristanians (and a perk for the cattle), for here it has attained perfection. The tubers are plant-ed out over several months to counter losses, and the potatoes are generally grown to excess, except in the meanest of stormy years. The potatoes are firm, creamy and delicious, and yet the patches are never rotated. The key appears to be the virtually disease-free volcanic soils, and the Tristanians' secret recipe: they plant the tubers with clumps of wool, rotted-down offal, and crayfish heads from the factory – the 'gearboxes' as the Saints would call them. Vegans might think twice before consuming a Tristanian potato.

Picturesque doesn't begin to describe the patches, which are blessed with names such as Red Body Hill, Old Pieces, Patches-on-the-Hill and Twitty Patch. Scattered between them are solidly built sea huts, more seaside chalets, used for storage of seed potatoes and tools but also as weekend getaways for fishing, drinking, barbeques and family frolics.

The Settlement Plain has in total some 1,100 acres of land, grazed by the main cattle herd and the sheep flock. Around the coast the island had three other livestock areas, accessible by boat in fine weather, which I would later visit: the Caves and Stony Hill on the southern tip, and Sandy Point on the eastern tip.

If I have gone into great detail, it is because the Settlement Plain encapsulates the Tristanian way of life. And because it was about to be violently changed.

THE FLOATING STONE
I had only been on Tristan da Cunha a week when the worst deluge in living memory struck the island.

In the wee small hours I was woken by the Big Watron angrily pounding boulders past my wall, and a commotion of heavy machinery somewhere nearby above. I crawled out of bed, hauled on some clothes and went out into the night. The Village turf was awash, the rain hammering down. The headlights of a digger flashed across a group of men in boots and waterproofs, holding shovels and mattocks, and beyond them was a raging brown torrent. The gentle Watron had gone berserk.

Martin Green, my then landlord and second in command at Agriculture, breathlessly acknowledged me. 'The Watron has burst her banks and is threatening to destroy these houses.'

'Is there anything I can do?'

'No, Joe. It's dangerous here. You could easily get swept away. The boulders are meat grinders. Go home and leave it to us. But thanks.'

Worse was to come. At the other end of the settlement, the Gulch was in devastating form. It isn't a spring: the Gulch receives its water from a series of waterfalls coming off a hanging valley way above. Only now it was loaded with the projectiles of five-, ten-, twenty-tonne boulders and an empowering cascade it could barely contain.

Daylight revealed the horrors. The gulch was now a small gorge and had greedily chewed away huge chunks of pasture and hurled them into the sea, where an astonishing new delta of rocks and boulders now fanned out from the beach. The digger's next task was to remake a way across the Gulch, and once it was passable, I walked out along the track to the Potato Patches. The track had been undermined and lifted, and in cuttings, completely buried, but the worst scenes were at the Potato Patches where thousands of tonnes of ash and cinder had washed down the mountainside and filled dozens of patches to wall height with a thick clayey sludge, entombing whole sea huts in the process. It was a mini Pompeii.

Reaching The Bluff, I turned round and walked back along the beach. Here too was a scene of devastation: sheep sheltering in the gullies that criss-crossed the Settlement Plain had been weighed down by their saturated fleeces, drowned and borne out to sea, then returned by the waves and dumped along the high-tide mark.

There was, though, one welcome discovery lying between the woolly carcasses, a rare talisman cast up by the now muddy sea. A floating stone.

The floating stones of Tristan da Cunha are lava anomalies, basalt bombs, a coarser form of pumice like big-bubble Aero, formed from undersea eruptions when the liquid magma hits the seawater and explodes into frothy rock; like the petrified head of a seismic cappuccino. They are highly prized by visitors and are famed for having had a transformative effect on the Tristanian community.

Usually, they are the size of tennis balls. This one was the size of a deflated beach ball, the colour of plain chocolate and beautifully contoured, the shiny, hemispherical interiors of the surface bubbles exposed by the sea's patient sculpting. Its tactility was addictive. I hurled it into the sea to prove a point, and the waves rolled it back to my feet as if to say: 'our work is done – it is yours'. And it is here now, by my side, as I tap away at my laptop and lay my hand on it to draw out the memory.

How did a stone that floats transform Tristan society? Connie Glass, the 'Rockhopper Copper', Tristan's policeman, filled me in. In 1975, Cunard's liner the RMS *Queen Elizabeth 2* called by, and the captain requested a couple of boxes of floating stones to sell to the passengers. The Tristanians obliged, and the money they received was put to buying the island's first TV and video recorder, which was set up in the library and became a new focus for weekend entertainment, showing the latest movies and opening their eyes to the modern world. It cemented a transformation that had already begun with the 1961 evacuation. As Harold Green told me, the evacuation, though terrifying and upsetting at first, had ultimately proved a good thing for the community. Not only did the Tristanians return from the UK with labour-saving appliances like fridges and irons, as well as the latest music and clothes from the debut of the Swinging Sixties, but with modified attitudes too. Under the colonial authorities, he said, it used to be a humble touching of the forelock and a 'Yes, sir. No, sir. Three bags full, sir.' After the evacuation, it was, 'You do your work and I'll do mine.'

ROOF RAISING

Lewis and I stood out on his front lawn with mugs of tea. It had become a regular habit in the evening when the sun was shining. He was deeply knowledgeable about the island and a good raconteur. I would hang on his every word, enthralled. From the raised position of the house, we could look over the whole east end of the Settlement, and the sea and harbour beyond.

'It's what we call a false lee,' he explained, waving his mug in an arc across the view. Throughout my childhood summers, my parents had sailed a much loved and leaky 1910 Falmouth Quay Punt called *Otter*, a gaff rigger, but in all our waterborne shenanigans I had never heard of a false lee. The wind was blowing hard, straight onshore, and yet there was something strange happening. It wasn't reaching us. 'Look,' he continued, now pointing with his other hand. 'All along the shore and some way out from the harbour, the sea is calm. Just a bit of bubble. Good enough for fishing. But look out further and to the east and west. Do you see the breakers?'

'Yes... yes I do. The sea's really rough. But how can that be possible?'

He turned and flicked his head up at the escarpment. 'It's the escarpment. It's pushing back. We're in a cushion of air trapped against the escarpment, and the wind is forced over the top. It's so high the cushion extends right out to sea. A false lee!'

There was no end to Lewis's stories. He told me about sailing in the longboats around to Sandy Point, where there was once a farming enterprise, to collect plums and apples from the orchards, and returning so laden that the gunwales were slopping over with water. About the curious place names, most famously Down-Where-The-Minister-Landed-His-Things, named for a cleric who was offloaded by ship in stormy weather, and – more in my line of work – the lovely Ridge-Where-The-Goat-Jump-Off. And about the day he took a longboat around the island to be astonished by a monumental, crewless oil rig grounded in the shallows. It was on its way to being scrapped and had broken its tow in a storm. It turned into a bonanza – the salvage company paid Tristanians to strip it down so it could be refloated and told them to keep what they could take.

'Next week we're going to replace the roof. It's quite an event, food and drink on me and Yvonne. Do you want to help?'

'Hell yes. Can I invite Dr Martin?'

'The more the merrier.'

As the only settlement in the whole Tristan archipelago, and far flung from the trappings of civilisation, the sense of community on Tristan is unparalleled. Everyone knows everyone, and everyone helps out. Sure, not everything is all sweetness and harmony, that's intrinsic in human nature, but disagreements are always put aside for the common good. It's survival.

When fish are caught and beasts are slaughtered, it's share and share alike. The old, vulnerable and disabled are looked out for. Generosity is universal. Often, I would find half a dozen freshly baked rolls on my living room table, or a prepared curry, or a few duck eggs, and one evening I recoiled in surprise to discover the indignant, glassy stare of a large, gutted fish lying across the bottom of my kitchen sink. Thanks to this strong community spirit, when help is needed for major projects or repairs, an All Hands Day is called, and the regular daily jobs are dropped for the task in hand.

Putting on a new roof is one of those communal events and celebrated in style. It mirrors the barn-raising of the Amish, with a twenty-first-century twist.

Come the day, the men gathered in the garden bearing armfuls of power tools, and the women poured into the kitchen with food, crockery and utensils. Soon the roof was swarming, as nails were pulled and the leaky tin was stripped off and handed down, the rain failing to dampen spirits or short-circuit drills. Meanwhile, in the kitchen, Yvonne choreographed the feast.

Lewis stood on the top of his gable like a magnificent finial, monitoring and orchestrating the process, and Dr Martin and I were soon helping to hand up the new sheets, which were rapidly shuffled into place, interlocked and pinned to the rafters. Buckets of cement were mixed and handed up to two Tristanians with trowels, who sealed off the gables and chimney breasts with mortar flashings even as the other end of the roof was still being laid. By early afternoon, the sun had come out and the job was done. Exhilarating teamwork.

On the front lawn Lewis had set out two long rows of chairs around a table groaning under bottles of drink, and indoors the kitchen surfaces were now obscured by bowls and plates of savouries, salads and desserts. The feasting was soon underway: generous and lethal 'Tristan tots' were downed to lubricate stomachs filled with delicious home cooking, and banter and laughter filled the evening air.

The division of labour might sound sexist to some – but it isn't. It is a joyful cultural event in which all present participate fully, a swift and efficient teaming of brawn and nourishment, and it works. That night I climbed under the blankets and slept snugly beneath a bright, fresh roof, delight-fully content.

RATTING DAY

Vets get asked to do some strange things during their career. But perhaps one of the strangest for me was to measure the length, to the last tie-breaking millimetre, of rats' tails.

On the Falkland Islands they have Peat Cutting Monday when Falklanders compete to cut the fastest, neatest slabs of peat from the peat beds. On Tristan they have Ratting Day, when Tristanians compete to cut the longest, scariest tail from the backside of a rat.

Ratting Day was originally an All Hands Day aimed at gaining some control over the pesky rodents that damage the potatoes and steal the eggs, but over the years it has turned into a day of competition and partying. Generous prizes are awarded for the greatest number of tails and the longest tail. And the splendid task of measuring the tails is given to the vet.

The rats, it seems, were introduced by one particular ship-wreck, and play havoc with the nesting birds. Which is why the Tristanians are forensic about checking their boats before motoring across to Nightingale or Inaccessible, both rodent-free and world-class seabird nesting sites.

Robin Repetto and Duncan Lavarello put their dogs Storm and Taz together to form a rat-hunting team and asked me along. We headed out on foot, weighed down with shovels and pick-axes, to the nearby pastures of Ginny's Watron and Bugsy Hole, climbing up onto the pediment of the escarpment where large boulders lay plentifully, half buried in turf, perfect capstones for rat hotels.

Catching the rats falls to the collies, and they revel in it. Storm and Taz rooted and snuffled around the boulders until they found a rat run, and then Robin and Duncan set to with the shovels to free the suspect boulder and lever it out with the pickaxe, the collies tensed for the pounce, eyes straining in gleeful anticipation. Often the rats would make a run for it, but fast as they were, the collies were faster. Execution was swift and efficient, a sharp bite and a quick, backbreaking shake.

Teams were scattered throughout the Settlement Plain, each targeting their favourite locations. Mouse tails were also included, and the loose-packed volcanic walls of the many potato patches were bedevilled with mice, so that teams targeting the prize for the greatest number of tails set dozens of mousetraps within the gaps between the stones, each marked with a little yellow flag wedged in the top of the wall.

Dusk, and the time for measuring was nigh. The teams gathered outside the bijou veterinary clinic, in truth a tired old hut next to Dereck's house, and Dr Martin, Dereck and I stood behind the consulting room table with gloves, a ruler and bags of seeping rodent tails. Drink was already fuelling a party atmosphere.

'You vets,' muttered Martin, screwing up his face as he emptied out the next bag of piss-covered tails, 'do the most disgusting things.'

'All in a day's work,' I countered, laughing agreeably. 'But I must admit, this takes the biscuit.'

And yet we still applied the medical acumen of the forensic pathologist to defeat the tricksters. In previous years there had

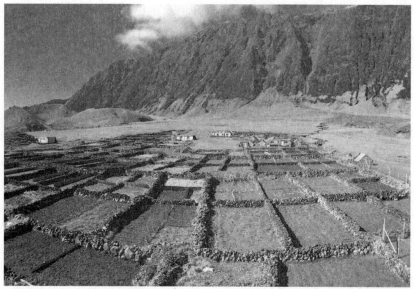

The Potato Patches

been an element of good-humoured skulduggery, with defrosted tails collected throughout the year being slipped in to boost the count, so we checked for the telltale signs of freezer burn and watery blood. And there was the blatant technique to encourage overmeasurement by slicing off a hunk of hairy buttock, but we had observed a useful final ring in the rat tail anatomy just post-anus which we adopted as our finishing line. Then there was the trick of stretching, so we palpated minutely along the full length of closely contesting tails to detect dislocations of the coccygeal vertebrae.

The results were in. Sean Burns, the Administrator, stood on the step with the liquid prizes.

'Winners of the most tails,' he announced, 'are Second Watron, with a total of 124 tails, an impressive 41.3 tails per person.' Roars of approval and raised drinks as bottles were handed out. 'A close second are the Coolers, a total of 68 tails, at 34 tails per person.' Another roar, more raised glasses and bottle handling. 'But the prize for the longest tail, the cream of the crop, goes to team Below the Hill, with a truly frightening 31.1 cm.' Whoops of joy for this hotly contested prize.

It was indeed an impressive and slightly disturbing tail, as thick as a whip. I asked Larry Swain, team leader, what its possessor was like.

'Huge – an absolutely huge boy rat about the size of a small cat with massive bollocks. Buck did well to tackle it.' He raised his drink. 'Extra dog biscuits tonight!'

Thank the Lord we didn't have to contest the bollocks.

DOGGY DOG WORLD

Two hundred and fifty islanders and one hundred and one dogs (no Dalmatians). About one dog per household.

Tristan has a large dog population, mostly working collies, because they are used for mustering the sheep and calves, and every household has a stake in the livestock. Each member of a household is allowed two breeding sheep, and each household, when I first arrived, two cows and followers (that is, the cows' offspring). Which rather neatly means that as soon as a baby bursts forth into sunlight, he or she contributes two sheep to the household flock. A birthing bonus, although probably not the first thing passing through the mother's mind. The father on the other hand...

I have an intrinsic love of the working collie. There are few greater pleasures than watching a dog work sheep at the command of its master, a canine ballet cum Olympian performance. Oddly, St Helena never developed this affinity with the loyal canine servant, and it often pained me to watch the ageing and arthritic farming community spread out over several hundred acres doing in an hour what a dog could do in ten minutes, instead of relaxing on one spot shouting commands while swigging coffee from a Thermos.

Every three months Dereck and I wormed and defleaed all 101 dogs in the tiny clinic next to his house, a veterinary marathon and a challenge for anyone wishing to retain a full set of fingers. But the modern flea products had worked a transformation on the island dogs, and the days of mangy-looking coats – in fact, flea bite dermatitis – had receded into the past, the flea seemingly banished. The most effective weapon was being able to treat all the dogs simultaneously, which is only possible because it is one village and everyone attends. There is no inhibition to pay because the veterinary services are free, financed by the islanders' communal pot of money earned from crayfishing, the core tenet of William Glass's utopia that lives on.

In a close-working agricultural community where the dogs intermingle, names become important hooks for command. I loved their variety, from the traditional Pip, Red, Hunter, Trigger and Fang, through to the more unusual Spinner, Watch, Number, Diesel and Trim. Of all the growlers and grumblers whose jaws I had to prise open, using, it has to be said, a vet's trick of pressing thumb on hard palate combined with speed, surprise and an occasionally brittle air of dominating confidence, there was only one dog that consistently defeated me. It was – of course, what other breed would it be? – a feisty little terrier called Popeye.

Paul Repetto, my shipboard companion, had become a close friend and he recruited me to join his lamb-marking team, a boozy tradition over several Sundays whereby the recently born lambs are chased down by dogs so that they can be sexed, marked, docked and if necessary castrated before rejoining the flock. Some dogs are obedient and soft mouthed, others are more atavistic and rip the skin, deaf to their owner's frantic bellows, and requiring my intervention with needle and suture.

The morning starts with a belly-busting breakfast sluiced down by beer, spirits, or in Paul's case, old brown sherry, and the team members take it in turns to cook. Come mine, I went for the traditional, whole hog, British farmer's breakfast of bacon, eggs, sausages, beans, tomatoes and fried bread, and presented Paul with a bottle of sherry I had relabelled 'Old Mrs Brown's Revenge'. It, and the breakfast, went down well.

Heavily fuelled in more ways than one, we then headed out into the sheep paddocks along with all the other household teams. I watched captivated, armed with my suture kit, as the many dogs were worked by their masters, some by shouted command with 'Come bye, come bye', others with peeps on their dog whistles, to target their ewes and pull down their lambs. The dogs interweaved back and forth along the pediments, each responding individually to their orders to isolate and pin down specific sheep. It is humanly impossible for us two-legged primates to chase down sheep on steep, bouldery terrain without breaking a limb or two, and the alternative of gathering them all up only loses the match between ewe and lamb. Instead, dogs take the strain and with wholehearted, doggy enthusiasm.

One stitch-up later – 'That dog's always doing that,' observed Paul. 'Vicious bugger!' – and we returned to Paul and Geri's for more victualling deep into Sunday evening.

To be repeated, week on week, until all the lambs were born and marked. The annual replenishing of the flock.

THE RECALCITRANT POTATO

'You're needed down at the crush.'

A calving, I thought. I grabbed the calving jack and rushed down the concrete track.

The cattle crush was in the small paddock just above the harbour, and I had already overseen several calvings there. My colleague Sue Harvey had visited previously and done a hugely successful round of artificial inseminations, using semen from world class bulls to boost the quality and productivity of the cattle, the only drawback being that sometimes the half-pedigree calves were a wee bit snug in the birth canal.

But a great advantage of artificial insemination is that the farmer knows to within a few days when the calf will be born. Close to their time, the expectant cows are brought into the Settlement and left in American Fence for observation, and it was my daily habit to walk through the graveyards on my way back to Lewis's, bid good evening to Corporal William Glass, and check for signs of labour.

But I wasn't being called to the crush for a calving. I was wrong.

It was a potato.

Eugene Repetto had forgotten to slice his potatoes, and his cow had swallowed one whole. Unfortunately, though, it was a gobstopper, a baking potato, and was now lodged in her throat. The bovine rumen is a fermenting chamber, and cattle have to burp or they bloat. The left side of his cow's abdomen was already ballooning and as tight as a drumskin. She was struggling to breathe. George Swain came to assist.

'George, see if you can push the potato towards me.' We had her head locked in the bale of the crush and roped to one side, and I had tied in a Drinkwater gag, a contoured wedge that locks between one set of upper and lower molars. Eugene meanwhile was battling to keep the head still. We managed to work the potato up towards the jawline, and the cow gave vent to a meadow-fragranced burp of such magnitude it virtually parted Eugene's fine head of hair.

But the whole process was fraught with danger. The bovine mouth is both long and surprisingly narrow, and my arm was in up to the elbow, rows of razor-edged molars threatening on either side to turn my fingers into pie filling. To push the potato down would risk a blockage in the chest over the heart, and that would kill the cow. Ideally, I would have used a probang, a concealed chopper in a long, flexible metal sleeve, and I could wish for one all I liked but the nearest was probably a few thousand miles away.

No. The damned potato had to come out from the front end.

'Push, George, push. I can feel it with the tips of my fingers.'

'I'm pushing, buddy, I'm pushing,' he gasped. 'But it seems to be jammed.'

It was. Behind the solid, cartilaginous block of the cow's larynx.

'I can't...' I was struggling. 'No, I can't get hold of it. It's too slippery. I can just feel the front.'

The smooth, spherical face of the perfectly round potato afforded no grip whatsoever, coated as it was in abundant, gloopy saliva. Added to which, every time I made the attempt I was closing the cow's epiglottis and asphyxiating her, which the 400-kilo beast responded to with understandable annoyance. Both Eugene and I were being violently jerked from left to right.

For an hour, a whole hour, I struggled to clear the potato, constantly re-jigging the gag to save my fingers as the cow worked it loose. Finally, I sat down on the grass and looked at George and Eugene.

'We have to rethink this before I lose my fingers.'

'What about some sort of corkscrew?' George suggested, thinking laterally. He was a smart, young guy who worked for Conservation.

'Good thought, George, but I just won't be able to handle it. There's no space in there. And anyway to be honest I think it'd just pull out. I have an idea though. Maybe we could go fishing. Give me ten minutes or so. I need to make something.'

I ran up to the Agriculture offices and threw a jacket off a wire coat hanger. In the toolbox I found the fencing pliers, and from the fridge pulled out a net of onions, spilling them onto the floor. I then fashioned a miniature landing net like a long-handled ladle, threading the onion netting around the wire loop to create a pocket and suturing it to size. I ran back down to the crush, reassessed the cow's mouth, and squeezed the loop into an elongated oval.

George beamed from ear to ear and nodded approvingly. 'I like it. A potato snagger.'

'OK, George. Gag in, potato snagger ready. Now... push against me.' I slid the snagger in over my fingers and wriggled it against the top of the potato, George battling to keep it in position as the cow objected. The snagger resisted, then with a palpable plop, slid forward and dropped down over the dome of the potato. I gave my improvised handle a sharp tug, and the potato flew out of the cow's mouth. It was an interesting variation on the Heimlich manoeuvre, bovinely done.

We cheered. I picked up the slimy potato and dropped it into Eugene's outstretched palm. 'Something for your dinner, Eugene. Parboiled.'

He slapped me on my shoulder with an impish grin. 'Thanks, buddy.'

'Oh, and Eugene. I'm going to buy you a potato chipper for Christmas.'

DENIZENS OF THE KELP

4.30 a.m. A calm day, a flat sea, a whisper of wind. A glimmer of light marked the eastern horizon. Cockerel crows and a barking dog resounded over the hushed village. I lay in the grass, waiting to see if the rumour was right.

Footsteps approached, and I sat up, startling poor Gary Repetto.

'Oh!' he exclaimed loudly, jumping backwards. 'I thought you were a dog.'

'It has been said! Sorry, Gary.' I let him recover his senses, and he leaned over to retrieve something from the deep grass beside the village gong, which was a tall, orange gas cylinder suspended from a wooden frame. It was a lump hammer. 'So, it's a fishing day?'

'Yes, we've had a long look at the sea and the sky, checked the weather online, and it looks good all day. Are you going out?'

'Horse and Wayne have invited me along.'

'Ah. Good fishermen. You should see plenty of crayfish. OK – prepare yourself. This is loud.'

Like a rural, scaled-down version of the Rank Organisation's trademark Gongman, he braced his legs and struck the gas cylinder a hefty blow. For a full four minutes Gary continued, blow after blow, and gas cylinder or not, its deep, prolonged boom resonated through the village as effectively as Big Ben stuck on midnight, stirring the residents and telling the fishermen to scramble from their beds, fill their flasks, and pack their sandwiches. I could even hear the nearby bell of St Mary's Church, reputed to be from the 1878 wreck of the *Mabel Clark*, pick up the vibrations and hum to its own monotonal tune.

'Don't you go deaf?' I asked him afterwards, but he didn't seem to hear me. I think it was a joke.

It wouldn't be my first encounter with this marvellous crustacean, source of Tristan's income. George Swain and Julian

Repetto had invited me to assist with a rockhopper penguin count over on Middle Island next to Nightingale, a distance of twenty-four miles, much like Dover to Calais. We motored out in Conservation's inflatable on a near perfect day, as it has to be for this potentially hazardous journey.

George explained how in the old days of sail, when Tristanians used the Italian-design longboats, the winds could change and trap them there for weeks. Once, two longboats were blown off course and missed Tristan altogether. They were thought lost before they clawed their way back over two long days to great jubilation. Often, the vessels were becalmed and the men were forced to row the twenty-four miles home.

Every day I walked past the last longboats on my way to work, now retired, upturned and battened down against the wind; ingenious lightweight, canvas-hulled, single-sail vessels that could be derigged, mast unstepped, tiller and rudder shipped, all in a trice so they could be dragged up onto the shore before being swamped by the surf. I would sometimes crawl under them and lie on my back, revelling in the brightly painted transoms and the craftsmanship of the local shipwrights. I once had the pleasure of interviewing former coxswain Lindsey Repetto, and he recounted the recipe for their construction, using local willow for ribs, mountain wood for elbows and knees, and shipwreck spars for mast, bowsprit, stem and stern. Refinements were made to create the fastest boat. It was customary sport to race each other back to Tristan.

This was the first time I had travelled far enough offshore to see the top of the island, the 2,062-metre Queen Mary's Peak, its remnant snow glistening in the sunlight. It took my breath away. The whole island stood proud on the platter of the sea, a perfect cone with a truncated brim like an Ottoman cap.

'I need to get up there,' I shouted to George over the roar of the outboard.

'Clive Glass is your man. He's an official guide. It's a long, steep hike. Some people do it over two days. You'll manage.'

Just before landing on Middle Island, George shot a few crayfish traps off the rock stack islet of Stoltenhoff. 'The best crayfish are over here,' George said. 'We left off fishing for a few years after the shipwreck. And they may even have fattened up on the cargo!'

On 16 March 2011, the MV *Oliva* drove hard aground in the narrow rocky channel between Middle Island and Nightingale. It appears there were no eyes on the bridge; at least no open eyes. In all the vast emptiness of the South Atlantic, this soya carrier collided with a tiny outcrop of volcanic rock.

The Tristanians rescued the crew with no loss of life. Human life, that is. But her fuel oil devastated the seabird colonies, despite valiant attempts by the islanders to de-oil and rehabilitate the penguins in pens and pools over on Tristan. Added to that, the cargo of soya soaked up the seawater, swelled, and mattressed the seabed, so it was largely assumed the crayfish had gone the same way. But crayfish are mobile, adaptable scavengers, and it's just possible that they, at least, thrived on the soya – a slim benefit. Because now they were huge.

I love a penguin. The Falklands made me fall in love with these hilarious waddling land creatures that turn into sleek, agile torpedoes. Rockhopper penguins are my favourite: doll-size, with red, angry beady eyes and a crazy spray of yellow feathers exploding from either side of the forehead. And they do what it says on the label: they rockhop.

After clearing the fur seals with shouts and long canes for fending off an attack – George had once been bitten in the groin and was understandably wary – I was tasked with counting rock-hopper nests. The nests were tightly packed, a colony of many hundreds on a rising slope, and I was to take a transect through the middle, counting as I went.

It had puzzled me why George and Julian were wearing welling-ton boots on the difficult terrain, covered as it was in slippery guano, whereas I, in my profound wisdom, had grippy hiking boots.

More fool me. As I worked my way up through the nests, deafened by the raucous braying, the rockhoppers leaned out to make their fury known by pinching my calves with their sharp, serrated beaks, as well as unravelling my laces in a cunning plot to trip me up and subject me to death by a thousand pecks. My count-ing aloud was punctuated with yelps and pleas for mercy. But for all my discomfort there was great beauty in what I saw: parents on eggs, and plump, fluffy chicks. And the colony was thriving again.

'Now I know why you wear wellingtons,' I called over to George in a strangled voice.

'I didn't want to say, but...'

I think the rest was lost to guffaws of laughter.

It was when we went back to haul the crayfish traps that I witnessed the seabed's generosity. Large and long, the Tristan traps are the most cunning I have ever seen, designed to cope with big catches. The bait is cleverly pocketed so that it defies consumption but continues to attract the crayfish, and one end is expandable with a billowing net like the belly of a miniature trawl that doubles the volume, but also allows the catch to be quick released into the bow of the boat with a quick tug of a purse-string cord.

I could hear the first trap straining the winch, the rope spurting seawater and whipping tight as it skidded along the gunwale. It was crammed with sixty or so crayfish, each at least half a kilo in weight, and often more like a kilo. In my youth I had made my own lobster pots and worked them off the Devon coast. A single lobster was a reason to celebrate. I had never seen or conceived of such bounty. The kelp forests off Tristan swarm with marching armies of crayfish, and in some of the purest, least polluted waters on earth. Barring shipwrecks.

Now, though, I was going to experience a proper working day in a crayfish launch with Wayne and Horse.

The seas down at Tristan, just a few degrees off the Roaring Forties, can be vicious and unforgiving, and there is no natural harbour, only the outstretched arms and the concrete wharves of Calshot Harbour which have had to be reinforced and rebuilt several times after storms. For this reason, the fishing fleet of nine launches are kept ashore on trailers and craned into the harbour when needed. I walked down to the quayside, which was alive with fishermen preparing their boats, and by 6.30 a.m. Wayne, Horse and I were motoring out of the harbour mouth.

The Tristan Lobster Fishery is harvested for crayfish – lobster and crayfish being synonymous but regularly muddled – under the auspices of Ovenstone, with annual quotas worked out locally by James Glass and his team. It's a shrewd move. Keeping the quotas in-house means there's less likelihood of plundering for short-term gains.

Across the four islands, Gough being the most distant at 255 miles away from the settlement, the overall catch usually amounts to more than 400 tonnes per annum, a highly valuable, renewable resource. The three offshore islands are fished by the company using their own fishing vessels but the waters off Tristan da Cunha are fished by the islanders. Suitable fishing days can be in short supply, though, and even with catches of three to five tonnes a day, the quota is sometimes missed. Then Ovenstone moves in with the big vessels to fill the gap. The islanders do their very best not to let this happen, and work hard to maximise their catches, creating an element of competition for heaviest catch of the day, and best lobster fisherman of the season.

Wayne and Horse had a plan. 'Usually we go round the island,' explained Wayne. 'But there's a reef just offshore from the Settlement that last year produced bumper catches. We'll drop our crayfish traps in a zigzag then work our drop nets along the coast and collect the traps before we go back into harbour this evening.'

The weather was perfect. We planted a long line of drop nets, simple baited rings, and pulled them all day, slowly accumulating the pinky-brown crayfish by their twos, threes and fives in the bow compartment of the launch.

Towards dusk we motored back to the traps off the Settlement. The factory horn had just gone, calling islanders down to process the day's catch, and we watched as some of the launches went in, but Wayne and Horse were having too good a day to throw in the towel just yet. Had the gamble paid off?

The first couple of traps were empty, but Wayne was not downhearted. As we worked our way offshore, the catches improved, although one trap was occupied by a large, replete octopus and fragments of dismembered crayfish.

'It's not always that way round,' Horse told me. 'They're old enemies. Sometimes the crayfish gang up and there's an octopus in the trap with no tentacles.' Nature red in beak and claw. Each on the menu for the other.

After that, the traps came up crammed. Wayne and Horse had hit the sweet spot.

In the now failing light, we chugged back into the harbour triumphant with nearly half a tonne of crayfish in the bow.

Wayne and Horse packed them into crates alongside the wharf before shackling the dangling chains of the crane to the bow and stern to lift the launch back onto its cradle.

I wanted to experience the last step in the process and so signed on at the crayfish factory, donating my pay to the pensioners' fund. 'Wear your rubber gloves,' Lewis Glass warned me. 'Crayfish may not have massive claws like your British lobsters, but their mouths will nip off the tip of your finger.' There's nothing like a pair of well-muscled, chitinous guillotines designed to rend flesh for trimming your fingerprint. I joined the tailing team, rapidly dispatching the crayfish and sending the fleshy tails along a water chute to a row of Tristanian women who then artfully removed the 'worm', the entrails, a skill that, even as a surgeon, I fumbled and never mastered.

At the top of the processing line, each crate was weighed and its contents checked to ensure none were 'in berry' – laden with eggs – or undersize, for which punitive fines awaited, then emptied into our stainless-steel trough, where Lewis would select the neatest, most vital and intact crayfish to go into the purging tanks instead of being de-tailed. These finest specimens would be cleansed of their intestinal contents over three days as they shimmied around in the tanks, then individually frozen intact and wrapped in gilded bags to be exported as valuable Japanese sashimi. They were allowed to have a maximum of one feeler and one leg missing (these kelp armies are always at war and play viciously) and to make up any marring deficiency a box of spares was kept so that the missing item could be replaced loose in the bag, for the benefit of the chef finessing his plate.

The factory is EU approved and as a veterinarian used to monitoring EU fisheries I was shown around the whole process. I was impressed. It was immaculate, a slick, well-conceived operation. From seabed to consumer, Tristan delivers a quality product internationally, a delicious crayfish grown in cold, healthy seas a long way from any discharging rivers or dirty land-masses. That, for a crustacean keen on scavenging – and when you think about the vile matter we pour onto our continental shelves – is thoroughly reassuring.

And the key ingredient for this tasty platter isn't some fancy mayonnaise. It's isolation.

A BAD YEAR

The winter bore on, never kind, but particularly harsh that year, and the cattle were suffering. My colleagues Sue Harvey and Aniket Sardana had begun good work on establishing mineral deficiencies in the livestock, and I intensified the programme, taking liver and serum samples and rushing them down to departing fishing vessels to be analysed in a South African laboratory.

The results were startling. Free draining, acidic volcanic soils leached by heavy rainfall are among the worst for mineral deficiencies, but as the results came in, I was astonished that the cattle were even standing; seemingly, they had adapted to the clinically impossible. I had never in my career seen such low levels of not one, but several vital minerals, and in synchrony. Copper, selenium, magnesium and in the sheep, zinc, were all well below the bottom end of normal, and each deficiency was in its own way potentially fatal.

A lack of copper, so important for fertility, was doubtless damaging the productivity of the herd and could be seen in their discoloured coats and spectacled eyes. A deficiency of selenium, an important antioxidant, causes extensive tissue damage and sudden death in growing animals. And magnesium. That's the brutal one.

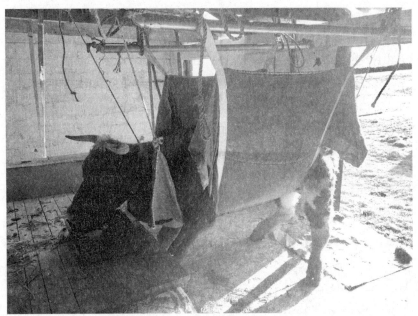

One of Tristan's downer cows recuperating in the sling

Magnesium deficiency provokes muscle tremors and sudden death through cardiac failure, but a nasty side effect is aggression in even the most benign of animals. Once, in St Helena, I had narrowly avoided death or mutilation on a farm at Fairy Land while checking a cow that was twitching and spasming. She gave me a hard stare from some thirty metres distant as we stood on an absurdly steep pasture studded with rocks. I shouted up to the herdsman and Rico Williams, my veterinary assistant, that it was undoubtedly magnesium deficiency and liable to be fatal. For whom exactly was about to be decided.

Suddenly she was head down and charging, but drunkenly, like a puppet having its strings jerked by a nervous puppeteer. I stood my ground and waved a token branch, but her gathering speed and the wet, steep slope that defied a rapid escape in my muddy boots could only result in one outcome. I braced myself for the impact of a 400-kilo battering ram in complete philosophical acceptance.

My branch shattered into several pieces as the cow and I became one tumbling projectile. All I remember is her weight as we shot down the slope, the cow using my body as a toboggan, narrowly missing all the projecting rocks that would have gouged me to ribbons. This brush with annihilation came shortly after I had nearly been shot while culling ducks in a forest, and rammed against a diveboat by a multi-tonne whale shark, a freak accident by a benign creature with poor eyesight that would have pulped me had she struck square on (though I did experience the unique joyride of being rolled down the full length of her back). Then there was the incident with the somersaulting bull... But I digress. That cow, as predicted, was dead by the evening.

So, the horrendously low magnesium levels in Tristan's pastures were not only killing animals but threatening safe handling. My colleagues had begun to remedy the situation with boluses, heavy mineral bullets that are pushed down the gullet of each animal and sit in the rumen, slowly dissolving and releasing goodness over months. I modified the type they were using and with my worthy team from Agriculture, particularly Riaan Repetto, who had to grapple every single slavering mouth and whom I would later mentor on St Helena, we bolussed all the sheep and cattle, a massive task. I also shipped in a pallet of salt licks and strung them out over the paddocks.

In due course the bolussing would have a transformative effect on the livestock. But in the meantime, we had a Tristan winter to get through, and the depleted animals started to succumb to the wet and cold, the damage wrought by the mineral deficiencies and the wretched parasites. They had colossal infestations of intestinal worms, and lice – which believe it or not can kill by causing iron deficiency anaemia. I had a battle on my hands, but with multiple enemies on all fronts.

The central issue was that we were overstocked for winter grazing, when the grass all but ceases to grow and gets cropped to its roots. Despite the noble efforts of Tristanians, driving out in the evenings to call up their animals and feed them potatoes, the cattle began to challenge me with one of the worst logistical headaches: downers.

Downer cattle are my personal nightmare. A 400- to 500-kilo beast crushes its own muscles, and unless it is put in a sling within twelve hours or so, the vet is on a long hiding to nothing. If the animal is down because of a tight calving, or an acute mineral deficiency caused by milk let-down, then it has a fair chance in a sling. But the truth of the matter was, I knew that these animals were doomed. They were, nutritionally and physiologically, in the end stage, and there is no coming back from that. But what vet shrugs their shoulders and does nothing? It would not have inspired confidence in the Tristanians who looked to me for answers. So, I tried and I tried, living a lie, each downer disheartening me further with the sheer futility of my efforts.

First, the patient had to be rescued in the bucket of the digger and brought into the Settlement. I manufactured a sling by redesigning jumbo harbour bags, rigging ropes and using cargo ratchets to hoist the animal upright from the beams of a small barn in the crush paddock. I pumped them with minerals, offered them food, applied salves to their sores, drenched them with fluids, all wholly supported by willing Tristanians, but to no avail. Of the nine I dealt with, not one survived.

Then there was New Zealand flax, both friend and foe.

On St Helena I had learned something useful about cattle and New Zealand flax. The island's peaks of cloud forest are blanketed with New Zealand flax – sadly to the detriment of the many endemic species – for the simple reason that it was once her monoculture. The Saints used to harvest the flax and bring it down by donkey to the numerous flax mills where the long fibrous leaves were defleshed in the scutching machines and processed into rope and string. In fact, St Helena had the contract for the British Post Office, and it was only the advent of synthetic string that caused her economy to collapse and the mills to fall into disuse. But it was well known that the waste from the flax mills fattened cattle beautifully.

In 2013, St Helena was afflicted by a severe drought. For the cattle pastures, where of course we would never turn off the water troughs, a drought is really a famine. The pastures parch, yellow and die; the animals starve. St Helena is blessed with a host of fodder trees, such as spore, olive, thorn, willow, acacia and loquat; we lopped their branches and fed them to the livestock, usually bundled up and tied with strips of the abundant flax. But as the drought wore on, the accessible fodder trees were stripped. I approached Andy Timm about feeding flax.

She liked the idea. But the long, lignified cords of the flax leaves can't be chopped by teeth alone. I had seen cattle chew a whole leaf, drawing it in like slow spaghetti, then spit out a ball of twine that wouldn't have looked much out of place on a stationer's shelf. 'You know we have the last chaffing machine?' she enthused.

I didn't, not least because I had no idea what a chaffing machine was.

The last chaffing machine was locked up in a shed over at Farm Buildings, and Gary Stevens not only had the key, but the sheer courage to operate it. It was a machine from the Devil's butchery.

Three scalpel-sharp machete blades were set flat into a large disc, spun at eyewatering speed by a long, whipping drive belt attached to an antique Lister diesel engine. Gary had to push bundle after bundle of cut flax down an ornate wooden chute dating from the 1930s, feeding this hungry maelstrom of blades, which he did with his usual bonhomie and a good dollop of tentative skill; the machine would have quickly turned his ham-like hands into finely sliced prosciutto. In this way, we created trailer-loads of food for the cattle. Flax saved the day, at least partly.

The Tristanians had an inkling that cattle liked flax, because the village herd of milkers chewed on the wind breaks surrounding the houses, leaving long, tangled manes of string whipping in the wind. But the only additional fodder the islanders were properly aware of was a type of fern from the mountain, only it wasn't sufficiently abundant or accessible to solve the problem. So I took my St Helena lesson to heart, borrowed a chain-mail glove – since a fingerless veterinary surgeon is no surgeon at all – and used a machete to finely dice bundles of flax leaves on a handy driftwood log. I was a very slow chaffer, parsley being more my métier.

Bucket after bucket I took out to the main cattle herd, as they didn't have access to the village flax and so didn't know to trust it. And slowly they acquired the taste. A number of Tristanians, including Lewis, added it to the regular menu. I even sent off a sample to a laboratory in South Africa for analysis, and it confirmed what the Saints already knew from the flax mills: it was surprisingly nutritious and even concentrated some of the minerals the cattle needed. I tried it myself; it was bitter and astringent, certainly no salad ingredient. The cattle were welcome to it.

Despite all these efforts we lost nearly 10 per cent of the herd: a pyrrhic victory, if it was any victory at all.

Sean Burns, the Administrator, wanted to prevent this ever happening again. It wasn't the first time. Previous harsh winters had caused similar mortalities, and I stumbled across an archived report from 1901 – 1901! – that said the island was overgrazed and overstocked with cattle. It was historically engrained; the islanders spoke of it as a norm, an acceptance of nature's cruelty. To me, it was understandable adaptation, but trying to take summer stocking rates through the winter without the benefit of conserved fodders or winter housing was simply courting disaster. Enough was enough. He tasked Alasdair and me to put together a proposal to take to the all-powerful Island Council: that each household should have not two, but one breeding bovine with followers. The rule would not apply to the Caves and Stoney Beach on the south side of the island, where animals were released to fatten in the wild, so there was some room for leeway.

It was a hard sell and had been tried before. The Tristanians are natural crofters, tilling the land, fishing and rearing animals. They enjoy having livestock and in numbers, so some residents baulked at the restriction. But by presenting a sound scientific case and a lenient road map, we succeeded in turning the wise heads of the council. We altered the seasonal cut-off date for numbers and gave households two years to slaughter down their stock and reach the new allocation. The feedback from Tristan has been that this control on numbers, along with the mineral boluses, has improved the health of the cattle enormously.

Sometimes less is more.

A SHIP FULL OF BULL

'Bulls,' Neil Swain said, eyeing Alasdair and me with a twinkle. 'The new artificial insemination bull calves won't be ready to serve for a couple of years, so we need to import a pair of bulls to bridge the gap. And I know just the man. Klasie Loubser. Can you sort it?'

'How do we get them here, Neil?'

'Well... on the fishing boats, of course.'

This was a challenge fraught with nightmarish logistics. How do you transport two bulls over 1,500 miles of heaving ocean on an old fishing boat? The answer is: not easily. But this tall order would have been impossible without the diligence and ingenuity of Klasie Loubser.

Klasie turned out to be a big noise in the Aberdeen Angus community of South Africa; he was President of the Angus Society and owner of the Holvlei Angus Stud. I soon found him to be the most amenable and dynamic of farmers, underlined a hundredfold when matters went awry at the eleventh hour. As they always do.

We exchanged emails.

'What I have for you,' he emailed, 'is a pair of sixteen-month-old pedigree bulls, one red, one black. They'll serve well. Just let me know what you need from me for the export certificate, and I'll get my vet onto it as soon as.'

The Aberdeen Angus is a sturdy native breed of good disposition that matures well on grass and produces excellent, self-basting cuts of marbled beef. Native breeds are traditional breeds designed to thrive in difficult environments with little access to luxuries such as nutritional supplements, created by bygone farmers who bred from generation to generation until they achieved their goal. Supreme among them is the Aberdeen Angus, ideal for the conditions on Tristan da Cunha, which approximates the wilder parts of Scotland.

My first challenge was drafting a certificate with a gamut of tests and treatments to protect the biosecurity of the island;

to prevent the importation of diseases and parasites. Above all, of course, venereal diseases to which cattle too are prone. Alasdair and Neil set about liaising with Table Bay Marine, the agents in Cape Town, and Ovenstone, who operated the fishing vessels.

Klasie took to the challenge with gusto. We purchased a standard twenty-foot shipping container, and he set his men to work with cutting discs and welders to convert it into a double bull pen. Meanwhile, I worked out a testing protocol with Klasie's extremely competent and enthusiastic vet, Dr Isak Rust.

Everything went far too well.

The shipment was destined for my old ship, the plodding MV *Baltic Trader*, and the afternoon before sailing, the bulls were trucked to the dock along with the converted shipping container. That evening I received the dreaded email, the inevitable last-minute hitch.

'The shipping company says the container design is unworkable,' typed Klasie. 'They need a whole lot of modifications otherwise the bulls can't go.'

'But she sails tomorrow. Is it possible?' I replied.

'How about your other ship, the *Edinburgh*? I'm told she sails next week.'

I spoke to Sean Burns, the Administrator, about delaying the *Baltic Trader*.

'No, I'm sorry, Joe. We can't delay her. She's already late and the timing is critical to the fishery. And,' he added, 'I'm afraid they've told me the container is impractical on the *Edinburgh*. It's now or forget it.'

Two bulls on the dockside in Cape Town with nowhere to go, and the next sailing of the *Baltic Trader* three months away, too late for the breeding season. Disaster.

But Klasie came back to me. 'We're going to try to perform a miracle. We've got the welders here and we'll work overnight to change the specs of the container.'

And a miracle they performed. New central doors, the end doors spotwelded shut, and Mark 2 pens at each end with higher bars, which probably saved me from being gored later.

The modified container, complete with two bulls bedded on sawdust, was swung onto the deck of the MV *Baltic Trader* and affixed to the on-deck container brackets, and with 800 tonnes of cargo, a puppy and a passenger called Bernard, the cranky old ship set out on her ten-day voyage.

It would be easy to think: mission accomplished. Think again.

When the *Baltic Trader* dropped anchor off the Settlement, conditions were far from favourable. She was rolling heavily in a side swell. The cargo pontoons are capable of handling twenty tonnes, and are powered by two 150-horsepower outboards, but they are not gainly vessels; they are lumpy, stubborn, thick-headed rafts with a will of their own.

We went out on the pontoon and my Tristanian colleagues assessed the situation. It was touch and go, but they decided to try unloading just the bulls, the puppy and Bernard the passenger. The rest of the cargo could wait. And wait it did, for a week.

I wanted to board and supervise the welfare of the bulls. The coxswain did his skilful best to marry up the pontoon and the dangling rope ladder. I knew the drill, thanks to my tutoring in the Falklands, but as I reached for a rung, committed to taking the leap, the pontoon and ship lurched violently apart. I felt my balance go. A strong hand hooked into my lifejacket and jerked me back from the brink. I could have been crushed against the hull, but the Tristanians are sea wise and vigilant. They've lost their own; they read the dangers.

At next attempt I swarmed up the ladder onto the deck and eagerly took stock of the bulls.

They were magnificent, shining young examples of their breed. Klasie had done us proud. But the ship at anchor was restless in the offshore chop, yanking and yawing at her cable, and the bulls were getting equally agitated. The black bull had a degree of serenity about him, but the red bull was pacing back and forth, bellowing, showing the whites of his eyes and gauging the top rail for an attempted escape. A loose bull on deck would be carnage and could only end one way.

I soothed and cooed and tried to work my animal magic, which to some degree did have the desired effect. These young bulls were used to handling and needed human reassurance. But we were on the verge of the next trauma. The derrick was trying to fit the four chains to each corner of the container so that it could be lifted over the freeboard onto the pontoon. But the fretful motion of the vessel was flicking the long, suspended chains into a deadly cat-o'-four-tails.

'Joe! Watch out!' someone roared.

The four chains flew through the container door inches from my face and slammed against the ceiling in a horrific cacophony of sound, the whole container booming like a gigantic kettledrum. The chains vanished just as rapidly, and I pinned myself against the pen of the now frantic red bull as they flew back in again. I was caught between a rock and a hard place – to be gored or chain whipped. It was hard to decide which I preferred.

Finally, the chains were wrestled under control and secured, then the derrick operator had the next unenviable task of getting the container over the side on a pitching vessel, the crane now a titanic steel metronome swaying through some thirty degrees. The airborne container began to swing danger-ously, but the crew and the Tristanians fought back, heaving on a web of ropes passed through deck ringbolts, resembling the Lilliputians grappling with Gulliver's tethers.

Now, poised over the sea, the container spun around and, with a piercing metallic screech, jammed against the topside of the vessel end-on. I tensed, barely able to watch. But again, they fought it back and the derrick operator dropped it onto the tossing pontoon, just avoiding a heavy landing with his skilful braking and split-second timing.

A swaying derrick, a rolling ship, a windy day, a cavorting raft on a heaving sea, and a four-tonne container twisting on chains with agitated livestock inside: a far cry from unloading onto a rock-solid wharf.

I felt a hand on my shoulder.

'Iz good entertainment, non?' said Bernard the passenger, merrily. I gave him the death stare.

When at last with huge relief we craned the container into the crush paddock and cautiously opened the doors, both bulls bolted across the steep central dip and then gambolled and frolicked with sheer euphoria, their copper nose rings gleam-ing in the stormy light. A large crowd had gathered to watch, and there was an overwhelming feeling of joy at this rare spec-tacle. I wondered how we would calm the frisky, overwrought animals, but this was where the preternatural powers of Jimmy Rogers came in.

Jimmy, Dereck Rogers's brother, had been born deaf and mute. Sharp-witted, short, bearded and hard-working, he was part of the Agriculture team and possessed of a powerful and instinctive bond with animals. His gaggles of hens and ducks, with their broods of chicks and ducklings, were famous for their meanderings around the Catholic Church of St Joseph near his house, and he would never sell one if he knew it was for eating. He also painted, his naive art mainly depicting scenes from the past – hauling longboats with teams of oxen, gathering livestock, milking cows – and when I left Tristan, I was very moved when he thrust two rolls of pictures into my hands, which are now among my most treasured possessions. In essence, he was an extremely nice man.

And a bull whisperer.

Never, we were told at university, trust a bull, no matter how friendly. They will kill you in an instant. A bout of protective jealousy or even a playful flick of the head can smash a human skeleton like kindling. But it turned out Jimmy gave off an aura that lulled bulls into a state of benevolence. I would watch, electrified, as he approached them with buckets of feed and they sauntered up to meet him, some esoteric form of communication passing between them, whether it was body language or pheromones I had no idea. Jimmy and the animals were on a special wavelength, and it was a marvel to witness.

Cherished, nourished and habituated, the two bulls settled in well and went on to father whole new generations of cross-bred Aberdeen Angus cattle. A flush of fresh genes, and a little piece of Scotland that had Alasdair beaming from ear to ear.

We should have wet their heads with a malt.

THE PEAK AND THE PEELINGS

'How on earth will we get her out?'

'Aha.' Clive Glass held up a bulging shopping bag. 'Secret weapon. Potato peelings.'

Weak after a long winter, Clive's cow had got herself into a pickle. She was in the bottom of a steep-sided gulch, seemingly unable or unwilling to get herself out. Clive had been feeding her there for days.

'Really?'

'You see that skinny track clinging to the side? We have to lay a trail of potato peelings. She loves them. It's our best chance, otherwise she's going to die down there.'

We scrambled down the path, no more than a slim ribbon pecked out of the side of the gulch by exploring cattle, but it was long and steep with twists and turns. Clive offered the cow a handful of peelings and she wolfed them down. She was at least thoroughly tame. He then laid a trail to the beginning of the path, and she took the first few wobbly steps.

The cow was weak, her ribs and pelvis showing, and her every movement was measured and slow. And yet gradually, hoof by hoof, peeling by peeling, she began the long climb to safety. But we had a long way to go, and I could see her losing her balance and plunging headlong into the gulch, which would finish her. We were just over halfway when there was another problem.

'That's it.' Clive was shaking a near empty bag. 'The last of the peelings.' Only the peelings made her step forward, other-wise she would just stand mopishly staring into infinity, but now there was no turning back. Indeed, no turning at all.

'Not quite.' I went back down into the gulch. She was an inefficient peeling gatherer. I crouched down and, crawling back up the path on hands and knees, collected every single potato peeling she'd overlooked. Back at her head, I started to lay down an accurately spaced Morse code of peelings, no overlap, no generosity, exactly staggered so that each peeling magnetically drew her forward.

Even so she left a few. Clive and I worked in relay, collecting the ever-diminishing supply from her rear and leapfrogging them past her to lay them down like exquisite truffles just out of reach of her prehensile tongue so that she had to inch forward.

And pretty much on the ceremonial laying down of the very last peeling, she emerged from the path onto the flat pastureland. It had taken almost two hours, and the light was fading fast.

'Good job, buddy,' said Clive. 'Want a lift back?'

The gulch was some way out on the Settlement Plain near the broken cone of Hill Piece, and it was a charming walk. 'No thanks, Clive. I think I'll take the opportunity to enjoy the evening air.'

An hour later I crossed the Gulch, the western entrance into the village, past the incongruous city bus stop sign. A dark figure peeled away from the shadows and fell in step.

'Drink at the Albatross?' murmured Clive. 'I've not been to the bar for years,' he added, almost by way of compliment.

I hadn't really known Clive too well until a few weeks previously when he had taken Dr Martin and myself to see the Ponds. Tristanians have a tendency to use diminutive names. The Ponds are three silver-surfaced lakes in a chain of steep-sided explosion craters, gargantuan divots of beguiling depth and beauty near the rim of the 2,000-metre volcano – which is also laughably known as the Hill. The trek was tough and had established my credentials.

Clive was an official mountain guide. The Hill isn't to be toyed with and a guide was not just essential but compulsory; the routes few and far between, the ash and cinder riven by gullies and neck-breaking drop-offs, and the volatile weather liable to close in, hurl sleet, destroy visibility and disorientate. In the past, several hapless visitors have had to be rescued, and on one occasion a missing Administrator was recovered in the nick of time, injured and unconscious. Clive was one of the few who farmed a separate flock of wild sheep that thrived on the ferns cladding the lower slopes of the Hill, animals of a different breed and meat to the domestic flock on the plain below. By day, he worked as a paramedic at the hospital, but his joy was to be on the Hill, and he knew its mazes and traps, its vagaries and its treacheries intimately. Two thousand metres at 38° south can be lethal. He was the man to have by your side.

We supped our beers in companionable conversation. Close up, he looked to be of the classic Scottish, William Glass mould: fair, freckled complexion and powerfully built. In Teeny's opinion, when she finally met him, strikingly handsome. Well, I suppose in a fair light...

'Clive, I hate to put this on you, but I want to climb to the summit of the volcano before I leave. Will you take me?'

'The Hill you mean! Sure, buddy. We'll make it happen. But now's not the time. Wait a few weeks for the weather to improve. Towards Christmas.' Christmas being midsummer.

'I suppose you've been up there plenty of times?'

'Maybe fifteen or twenty. But you know, Leo my son has never been. We'll take him too. And Kash of course.' Clive would never go anywhere without his loyal companion. They were bonded at the hip. Kash was an exceptionally intelligent long-haired chocolate-and-white collie whom Clive adored and I too had come to love. I always joked with him that Kash was really my dog, and he was just the caretaker.

'And I want to swim in the summit's crater lake.'

'What?' Clive put down his beer with a thud. 'Oh great,' he said. 'That means I have to as well. Thanks a lot, buddy,' he added, good-humouredly.

I later sealed the deal with a bottle of Johnnie Walker whisky. 'Put it on the top shelf,' I told Clive. 'Not to be touched until we come down off that volcano. And I'll know if you've diluted it with cold tea,' I quipped.

And so, a solid friendship was forged by the unlikely means of a bag of potato peelings.

I couldn't wait to climb the volcano, as ubiquitous and invisible as a creator god from the Settlement but alluringly beautiful when seen from the sea, mantled in snow. And Clive had promised me a concealed wonder in the shape of the crater lake. But first I had a big birthday to get past. Lovely Geri Repetto, she of the chickenpox, had persuaded me to have a party to celebrate my sixtieth.

'I'm not really one for parties, Geri,' I had said, all bah humbug.

'Oh, come on, buddy. Tristan parties are the best and I love organising them. Leave it to me. Everyone will come, you'll see, and we'll get Clive to play the accordion.' Her generosity of spirit shone through.

I didn't regret it. It was the best party I've ever been to. Geri organised the food and drink and decorated the capacious community hall. Pictures from my veterinary career were plastered across a wall over trestle tables groaning beneath stacks of fragrant home cooking. The centrepiece was a cake, an ingenious artwork of enormous proportions embossed with pawprints and dog bones, and sprinkled with gaily coloured, icing medications, all looped within the coils of a surprisingly lifelike marzipan stethoscope.

I had specifically put on the invitations, 'Please don't bring presents. Just bring yourselves', but the giving of gifts is a powerful Tristan tradition that cannot be denied. As the hall filled, each new arrival approached me with a package, and by the end of the evening I had accumulated twenty-three pairs of many-coloured hand-knitted woollen 'love' socks, whose rings of vivid colours had in the past been used to coyly convey messages of affection,

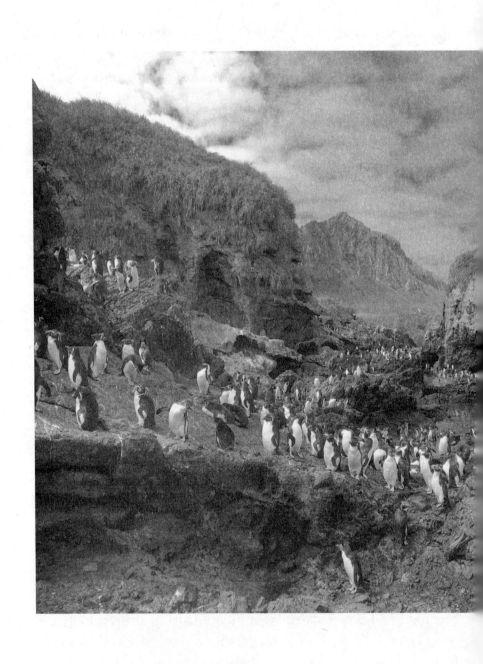

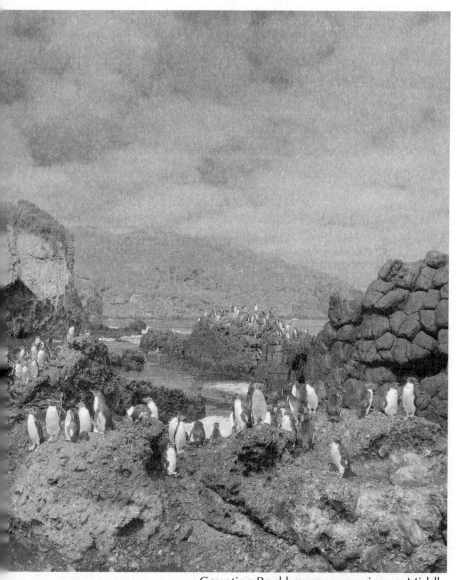

Counting Rockhopper penguins on Middle Island, Nightingale, Tristan da Cunha five hand-knitted sweaters, seven woollen beanies and an array of keyrings, bottle openers and deodorants.

Towards the end of the evening, party in full raucous flow, Clive pulled out his squeezebox and struck up the notes for the Pillow Dance. The floor cleared and the hall fell silent as he billowed his instrument back and forth, filling the air with jollity.

A small pillow, embroidered with a longboat, was thrust into my hands, my task, to select a lady from the now seated partygoers, drop the pillow in front of her, kneel, and give her a peck on the cheek. I picked on pony-tailed Nessie Lavarello, my daily supplier of coffee and fresh milk, and then attached myself to her hips in the beginnings of a conga as she danced across the room to lay the pillow before a chosen man and repeat the process. The children decided to start their own snake, and as the accordion played on, two long congas grew and coiled and collided around the room, to much well-oiled laughter. In former times, and maybe even now, this ritual dance gave shy young islanders a way to indicate their favour. It is a dance steeped in old-world charm and, I believe, uniquely Tristanian.

Clive followed through with the Donkey Dance, Shottee, and John Piddliwigg. Thanks to Geri and the cheery participation of the islanders, it was an evening to treasure. At some ungodly hour I gathered up my bounty and staggered back to Lewis's place.

Producing knitwear, as in the Scottish islands and the Faroes, is a deeply embedded crofting tradition. The Tristanians are adepts, and there is rarely a party, fishing expedition or trip to the beach where someone isn't clicking away with knitting needles using pure finger memory while in full-flow conversation. And although nowadays imported wool is often used, the complete, labour intensive, hand-creation from sheep's back to human torso is also still undertaken.

Shearing Day, an All Hands Day, is a pivotal social event held just before Christmas when the knitters of the island gather their fundamental necessity: the wool. The weather can be temperamental, but as it happened, my Shearing Day, where I was attending both as shearer for Paul Repetto's team and as vet to zip up any shearing nicks, was bathed in sweltering sunshine.

The whole community gathered above the Potato Patches at the Pens, a ramshackle, weather-beaten maze of planks, driftwood and pallets strapped together with posts and fencing wire to create a space for every team to draft out their sheep, drag them into a pen, and attend to their needs.

Paul handed me a pair of fiercely honed Sheffield steel handshears. I was a little rusty, even if they weren't. 'Try not to butcher her, buddy, and if you cut off her teats you can bloody well stitch them back on again.'

I grinned back – as befitted the day – rather sheepishly.

Meticulously, inch by inch, I relieved my ewe of her thick and heavy burden. It was like sculpting a new animal out of warm snow with my ever-softening lanolin hands. Her relief was tangible, and the whole tactile process deeply satisfying, even if Paul was shearing four sheep to my one. Once we'd finished and the barbecues were sizzling, Paul passed round a bottle of crème de menthe, which for some obscure reason, taken in medicinal glugs, tasted more like a reviving elixir than the customary toothpaste.

Outside the pens a row of women sat chatting in picnic chairs, clicking away with their knitting needles, several with cumulus clouds of rolled fleeces around them. Occasionally one would lurch forward to lay claim to a particular fleece with a choice shade of brown or black. These select fleeces would then be picked clean of debris, carded, spun on home-made spinning wheels, coiled into loose skeins, washed and hung out to dry.

My chocolate-and-grey, ribbed-and-cabled Tristan wool sweater is the snuggest thing in winter and beats synthetics hands down. One of the greatest – and sneakiest – advertising coups of the synthetic clothing industry was to steal the word 'fleece', but they can never steal the quality.

The weather stalled my conquest of the summit several times, but finally, a week before Christmas, the day dawned still and cloudless. Even the sea was in bed, the horizon crisp and sharp, visibility at its keen-edged best. Clive, Leo, and I – not to forget enthusiastic Kash – took the first brisk steps up the sloping pediment in the purest of early-morning sunshine.

At 800 metres we crested the escarpment onto the Base – the lower vegetated slopes – and paused to take in the bird's-eye view of the Settlement directly below, now awake and setting about the day. All around spread an entirely new landscape of thick fern bush, with here and there the flash of a magnificent Atlantic yellow-nosed albatross sitting high and mighty on its throne-like pedestal nest, sometimes with a downy chick. It was a captivating world, fresh and alive.

Higher up, the cone took on a meaner aspect, loose cinder and shards of magma skittering under our toiling legs as we ascended higher and still higher, until finally we came to the rim of the mother crater, the peak itself. My Hillary-Tenzing moment.

Clive took a dramatic stance and held me back. The crater rim is sharply defined, an almost perfect cup of shattered, Mars-red rock, except for a smooth depression, like the pouring lip of a gravy boat.

'This is it, buddy. When we go through this dip you'll see a wonder of nature.'

It was the crater lake: deep, lucent, vitreous, and by some magical collusion of sunlight and algae, sparkling with gold and emeralds. It was also, through a whim of the last eruption, a perfect heart shape. A genuinely breathtaking spectacle.

While Kash tore back and forth, we walked the rim, marvelling at the views untrammelled by cloud or mist and spying out the features on Tristan's coastline. We came to a stop at a small cairn with a rotting flag that marked the highest point. Clive crushed my hand.

'Congratulations, buddy, you made it. Queen Mary's Peak. 2,062 metres, 6,765 feet. And all of Tristan beneath us.' He turned to Leo, and with barely concealed pride added, 'Well done, son. Now, there's a small painful matter of a crazy deal we made.'

We ran down the crater's inner scree slope to the water's edge, and with howls of masochistic pain, threw ourselves into the heart-stoppingly cold waters of the glittering lake, then laid out on thick beds of spongy moss to recover and dry in the unalloyed sunlight.

'Time to get back down,' said Clive reluctantly, heaving himself up from the comfy moss. 'But first, a traditional ceremony to perform.' He went down to the lake's edge and filled his empty bottle with crater water, then raised it like a flaming torch. 'For the whisky!' he proclaimed, with feigned gravity.

Back down in the Settlement after a skidding, sliding, galloping descent, Clive fetched the bottle of Johnnie Walker off the top shelf and, cracking the seal, poured out generous Tristan tots with a dash of crater lake. Not a hint of cold tea. Clive's wife, Vera, had prepared a feast, and we all, Kash included, slipped into that utterly relaxed, dreamy world of complete and total contentment. Then Clive lifted down his accordion and wheezed out some shanties.

It was a day without compare: a great climb with grand views and in good company, sealed with an invigorating dip in a bejewelled lake of ethereal beauty. Undoubtedly my finest day on Tristan, and one of my finest days ever.

THE JOINING OF THE CIRCLE

Sean, the Administrator, handed me the lump hammer. 'Your turn, Joe. Give it a good whack.'

It was just past twelve on Old Year's Night, and a boozy crowd clustered around the village gong above the hall. Striking the gong is a sacred ritual confined to fishing days and emergencies. It is the village voice, a masterful clarion call-to-arms that rouses the whole settlement. To strike it frivolously is to cry wolf, a blasphemy liable to invite the deep disapprobation of the Island Council, the ripping off of epaulettes and the shameful banishment back into the frothy turmoil of the outer world.

But at the turn of midnight on Old Year's Night, anyone can have a go. It was with great pleasure and a slight loss of hearing that I gave the orange gas cylinder an almighty ringing blow sufficient to make Corporal William Glass down in American Fence stir in his long repose.

The Tristan community take a month's break over the festive season, and by Old Year's Night everyone is fully relaxed. Throughout the day the village had been in party mode, and groups of ghoulish monsters, the Okalolies, islanders fully togged up as fiends from the very worst of nightmares, swarmed from house to house to chase away the devils of the old year.

Everyone, Okalolies and all, wound up at a garden party at the Administrator's residence, and the festivities rolled on beyond midnight.

My time on the island was drawing to a close. I had always intended to retire at sixty, and Tristan was to be my last hurrah, the destination I would never reach, but did: the perfect culmination of my veterinary career. Fate, though, had its own ideas. An unprompted email turned up in my inbox from Darren Duncan on St Helena.

'How are you fixed after Tristan? Cat Mann, the vet who replaced you, is returning to the UK to have a baby. Do you want a job?'

And then, as if to convince me, an old friend changed her itinerary at the very last minute. It was Alasdair who broke the news. 'Did you hear, Joe? The RMS is on her final voyage and has decided to divert to Tristan for one last nostalgic visit.'

'You're kidding? So, if I'm going back to St Helena, I won't have to take a fishing boat to Cape Town after all. I can go direct. Perfect.' It was uncanny good fortune.

When the familiar mustard funnel of the RMS hove into view and dropped anchor offshore, I knew the circle was to be joined. Typically, it was too rough for the passengers to land safely, but after many hugs and last-minute gifts on the wharf I was taken out to the ship on a pontoon. In a tricky manoeuvre and during a momentary lull between waves, the ship's derrick hooked on to the 'air taxi' – a metal coffin – and flicked me on deck as if landing a mackerel. Now I knew how the bulls felt.

The ship was packed with Saints and tourists, all keen to experience the last true Royal Mail Ship's final ever voyage, the end of a maritime tradition. Teeny was among them and there to welcome me on board. It was a homecoming.

The winds kept up their agitation of the sea, and Captain Adam took the RMS over to Inaccessible Island, there to seek shelter beneath her daunting cliffs, ribboned with Tolkienesque waterfalls. So densely packed with nests is this World Heritage Site, so criss-crossed is the sky with seabirds in flight, that at nightfall a curfew was enforced and all superstructure lights extinguished to prevent the decks from being covered in feathered confusion.

The passengers made it ashore on Tristan – for three hours. A mutinous group of probable landlubbers who failed to under-stand the impassive appetite of the sea had badgered poor Captain Adam, who then skilfully worked out a compromise. Fit and able passengers were harnessed and lowered down the ship's ladder one by one into a waiting inflatable and a nest of powerful Tristanian arms. I took Teeny ashore where she was ladled with gin and Clive drove us out to see the Potato Patches. But it was a strangely disjointed day because my fine friend Trevor Glass, Lewis's eldest son and the man who had lured me to Tristan, had very tragically lost his wife to an acute illness just the previous night. When the island loses one of its number, the whole settlement goes into mourning. I felt, in a way, that we were treading on their grief.

After three hours, Captain Adam gave three long blasts on the ship's horn that rattled the settlement and bellowed, 'Return now or be marooned', and passengers trickled back to the waiting inflatables. At the quayside, Geri, Paul and Neil were there to see me off for a second time.

'See you again, buddy.' Neil crushed my hand.

Geri gave me a warm hug and pressed another pair of hand-knitted woollen love socks into my hands. 'In case you run short,' she said. I burst out laughing.

Paul thumped me on the shoulder. 'Now this time bugger off,' he joked.

Teeny and I exchanged glances. She'd been pulled into Tristan's heart, and there was no doubt that for all the bravado we both looked emotional.

A pair of strong hands reached up and lifted Teeny bodily down into the bucking inflatable. Larry Swain, winner of the longest rat tail. I leaped into the bilge and sat beside her on the sponson.

'Teeny,' I murmured in her ear. 'I'm going to miss these people. None better on god's earth.'

'Yes,' she replied simply. 'None better.'

DOORSTEP CORNUCOPIA

The last mail ship on her final voyage. It was a historic occasion that I wanted to be a part of as the RMS had so massively been a part of me. For St Helena, too, it was like the passing of a family member, and the island laid on a fortnight of celebrations. I made arrangements to return via the new airport, and stayed aboard for the final leg to Cape Town, a voyage of commemoration, of feasting and cocktail parties, of ship's crew cabarets, of Captain Adam's marathon 'gin for Jesus' after the last shipboard Sunday service, and of the auctioning off of company flags and Post Office pennants, until the final silencing of the engines in Duncan Dock at Cape Town drew genuine tears all around, as if we'd killed a favourite aunt. She was to be torn apart, scrapped for her organs.

However, there were a couple of final twists in her tale. In the end, she wasn't scrapped. She was initially repurposed to carry munitions for the anti-hijacking patrols through the Indian Ocean, an ignominious fate. And then she was entirely reincarnated as the fully refitted St Helena for Extreme E, a 'floating paddock' carrying VIPs and off-road electric racing cars to championships around the world, the future of motorsport. She lives on, and with dignity.

Several months after my return from Tristan to St Helena, firmly re-ensconced in my former role, the indefatigable bio-security officer Julie Balchin chased me down at the office. 'You'd better get back home quick. You've got a crisis.'

'Oh no, what's happened?' I asked in alarm, fully expecting to hear the fire brigade were hosing down the smouldering ruins. She had just returned from checking passengers alighting from the cruise ship the MV *Plancius*, up from Tristan.

'Go and see.' She winked conspiratorially. 'And if you can spare a few...'

I rushed down to the house. My front door was barricaded.

Unbelievable. Five bulging feedsacks of Tristan potatoes and two large cases of frozen lobster tails.

Those amazing Tristanians...

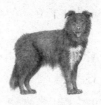

ROSIE AND THE FRIAR

Blind fear, that seeing reason leads, finds safer footing than blind reason stumbling without fear. To fear the worst oft cures the worst.

Cressida in Troilus and Cressida, Act 3 Scene 2

TRINITY

This is a story about a dog, a beekeeper and a stone giant.

THE STONE GIANT

Every morning, while I have the pleasure and privilege of staying at Sydenham House, one of the limited collection of heritage buildings owned by the government called, oddly, the Chief Secretary's Houses, I drag myself from under the duvet and draw back the curtains onto a lush, tropical garden. Cork oak, rose apple, avocado, pecan and rubber trees jostle for light over flowerbeds crowded with agapanthus, red hot poker, cape gooseberry, frangipani and an array of assorted succulents. The lawns have been further ornamented by some heritage kleptomaniac with a massive sea anchor, cast iron horse troughs, trypots and heavily toothed cogs from a flax mill. Beyond, a backdrop of the dry coastal lowlands – the Crown Wastes – falling sharply away to a broad Atlantic horizon.

In the middle of this pleasant scene rears the dinosaur-backed ridge overhanging Lemon Valley, its spine of tumbled volcanic rock like a topping of crushed biscuit. It is fierce, sheer sided and unforgiving. And in a little dip on this brutish wall and central to my view stands a defiant figure, tall, angular and impossibly misplaced in this realm of fractured chaos: The Friar.

I never did understand gravity. Friar's Ridge, with its loose and rotten scatter of shattered rock piled along a knife edge like a deranged linear Jenga, is hideously dangerous and seems liable to tumble into the valley at a moment's notice. And that is why The Friar, an improbable natural tower of rocks teetering on this knife edge, is extraordinary.

I had a fixation with The Friar, which as it turned out, was fortuitous.

There is an obscure branch of seismography that studies PBRs, precariously balanced rocks, those geological wonders that have somehow resisted millions of years of erosive forces bevelling out the landscape all around and reached an unlikely equilibrium with gravity.

Some bright spark of a geologist was having a think over a peanut butter sandwich one day when the light dawned that certain PBRs could not exist if there had been any significant recent tectonic activity. Recent, as in the past few centuries. When it comes to building a dam or nuclear power station, or perhaps – and why not? – a cloud-tickling pagoda, this is invaluable information.

And it gets cleverer. The trick is to look back in time. Rocks, believe it or not, sunbathe and get the equivalent of a tan. They are bombarded by cosmic rays which convert oxygen atoms into beryllium-10. These accumulate and can be counted. By creating a three-dimensional model of the PBR, with its layers and components, its age according to B-10, its density, centre of gravity, mass and stability, and throwing the whole set of ingredients into a cunning algorithm, it is possible to say there has not been an earthquake of 'x' magnitude in the past 'y' millennia. So... go build your record-breaking pagoda.

For this reason, PBRs are called inverse seismometers, or in more friendly terms: rock clocks.

The Friar is St Helena's outstanding PBR.

The reassuring thing about The Friar is it is so absurdly precarious that it just shouldn't be standing. We can dispense with the cunning algorithm and truly say that St Helena, the volcano, is retired from active service – extinct. Unlike Tristan da Cunha, which was thought to be extinct but, as we have seen, blew its nose rather spectacularly in 1961 just a stone's throw from the Settlement. Anything more than a frisson of a rock tremble would have sent The Friar diving headlong into the valley long ago.

The reason is the Mid-Atlantic Ridge, that 10,000-mile-long divorce settlement between vying tectonic plates as the Old World and the New World tear apart from each other. It is the longest mountain ridge in the world, submerged and hidden from view bar its highest peaks, a chain of beautiful islands from Iceland and the archipelagos of the Azores and Cape Verde, to Ascension, St Helena, Tristan da Cunha, Gough and into the deep-frozen south to Bouvet.

St Helena was born on the ridge, a violent birth of explosive magma and toxic gases forcing a path through the 5,000 metres of overlying ocean to blister up some 1,500 metres into the open sky. Eight million or so years of erosion since dormancy have reduced the height to a humble 823 metres, so the dramatic scenery, including The Friar, are the exposed remnants of her once fiery mouth. The divorce is ongoing, and inch by inch, year by year, the Atlantic shoves St Helena deeper into retirement.

She now lies over a hundred miles off the active zone, and frissons are about all she receives.

Despite the spine's vertiginous flanks, I was told that it was possible, with some care, to reach The Friar, yet it seemed that in these modern times few Saints are inclined to bother and none I asked knew the way. But my daily vista of this colossal, monkish figure was irresistible. Ted, our incumbent agronomist, was a serious technical climber on both rock and ice, and lived in the vale just below. I asked him.

'Yes, I often go up there in the morning before work. The scenery is stunning, and the other side plummets vertically into Lemon Valley. Come off the ridge when it gets dangerously narrow and follow the contours on the side. You'll find they work their way up to the dip, and The Friar sits on a small saddle of rock.' He shook his head. 'I thought about climbing onto his head, but it's so precarious. You can see right through him! I'd have died for sure. Oh and – take care. The whole ridge is rotten. Don't go too close to the edge or you're strawberry jam.'

Strawberry jam. My preference was cherry. But those words were to resound in my head some time later.

I set off, armed with a machete. I first walked down into the adjacent valley of Guinea Grass, past the community hall and into the almost impenetrable scrub and prickly pear below the housing, where a ruined cottage slumbered abandoned and forgotten on the edge of a dry waterfall. At the end of the overgrown track, I found someone had cleared a plot and felled the fir trees. I crossed the clearing and climbed up onto the ridge, at first manageable rectilinear blocks of basalt pierced by starved, truncated scrub, then narrowing into less comfortable broken teeth with nasty drop-offs. I scrabbled back down onto the steep flank of the ridge, gripping branches and clambering over spiky fallen trunks, seeking secure routes through and around the jutting fists of rock. Eventually the vegetation thinned, and sure enough, just as Ted had said, the rock face became a series of ledges running obliquely up to the dip on which The Friar stood, now out of sight somewhere above me.

And then I was there. The Friar, from a distance so diminutive in the wide, open landscape, was now hulking, a strange and monstrous tor of counterbalanced rocks that patently defied the laws of gravity. Above its solid pedestal, the whole mighty tower was cleaved into blocks so eroded that bright oceanic light shone through the joints off the Atlantic beyond. It was as if The Friar had been hastily erected by some bored, lunatic god who had no concept of balance but struck lucky. Narrow at the base, broadening over the belly, with a humped back shouldering a loose cowl and topped by a head with a jutting chin, it was an almost ridiculous assemblage of lichen-embossed boulders, but all the more awesome for that. Especially as everything around looked as if it had been trashed by a wrecking ball. I could only assume that a whim of erosion had counterbalanced its component rocks. The small platform that surrounded the pedestal, though, was solid and secure, fit for a spectacular picnic.

I relaxed and savoured the surroundings as the rock began to bronze with the sinking sun, and then, hugging the pedestal of The Friar, craned my head gingerly over the far edge. A vertical wall dropped into the deep, V-shaped gorge of Lemon Valley far, far below. Pure death. No clemency. Cherry jam indeed.

THE DOG
It was the 4th of January, a Monday, and we had just come back to work after the Christmas break.

'We have a missing dog.' Ken put down the phone. 'Tony Leo's dog, Rosie. He's away on medevac and Rosie was being looked after by his brother. On New Year's Eve, someone let off fireworks half an hour early from High Knoll Fort, and he lives just below. Rosie went crazy and bolted.'

Tony Leo was the doyen of beekeeping on the island and had been chairman of the Beekeepers Association for many years. He was deeply knowledgeable about the hairy little honeymakers and was both engaging and eloquent. He had also been one of my staunch supporters when I first came to the island and sang bass with me in the choir. I considered him a friend, and the fact that he was away in hospital made me all the more determined to track down his loyal companion.

Firework phobia is a common problem in dogs due to their acute sense of hearing and frequent failure to understand that the booms and flashes aren't really heralding a canine Krakatoa. I've known dogs to chew through doors in their panic.

'Does Tony know?'

'Don't think so. He's about to go into surgery in the UK, and they won't want to worry him.'

'I heard the fireworks too. I thought it was midnight and had to check the time. Damn things.'

'They knew she hated fireworks and were about to tie her up. There was one sighting later that night down at Rosemary Plain, and she was running.'

Rosemary Plain is a grassy common at the start of Friar's Ridge and a common party spot, but a long haul from the sprawling citadel of High Knoll Fort. She must have been running like the devil. 'But that's almost four days ago. Not good.'

Not long after, the phone rang again. Ken hung up with a knowing look on his face. 'Andy's parents, Joe.' Arthur and

Heather, my line manager's mum and dad, were long retired and lived with Andy's assorted collection of sheep, goats and chickens as well as a pair of superannuated turkeys that had never learned the significance of Christmas, all in and around a long, stone cottage that I had always envied. It perched on the edge of Crack Plain, an open palm of habitable land with a billion-dollar view over a plunging rock face that marked the head of Lemon Valley. Ken continued: 'Over the weekend they've heard a dog howling somewhere below in Lemon Valley, but they can't really say where.'

'That has to be Rosie. Just near the last sighting too. So she's not dead, she's trapped.' A human can barely go four days without water before slipping into a coma, and though dogs are more resilient, her time had to be running out.

Steel-haired and clear-headed, Heather sat us down in the animal-strewn garden and filled us in. A dog had been howling on and off for two days, but the sound was distant and the enormous rock walls of the valley simply ricocheted the noise all around, causing it to lose meaning and direction.

The term 'valley' is understated on St Helena. There are very few true valleys as would be understood by a lowlander. They are gorges, chasms and ravines. Directly beneath us the floor of Lemon Valley, a gorge, dropped rapidly and unrelentingly to the distant ocean and the complex remains of gun batteries and a maritime quarantine station where crews were once sent to live or die from smallpox and other shipboard plagues. The valley floor, the gut, is made virtually impenetrable by dense, inter-woven vegetation criss-crossed with fallen trees, but a narrow, giddy path threads down one side beneath Friar Ridge.

We fell quiet and strained our ears. Nothing. And then a single, distant, short, sad wail. Instinctively we all leaned forward as if to get closer to the source, but it was fruitless. Again, nothing.

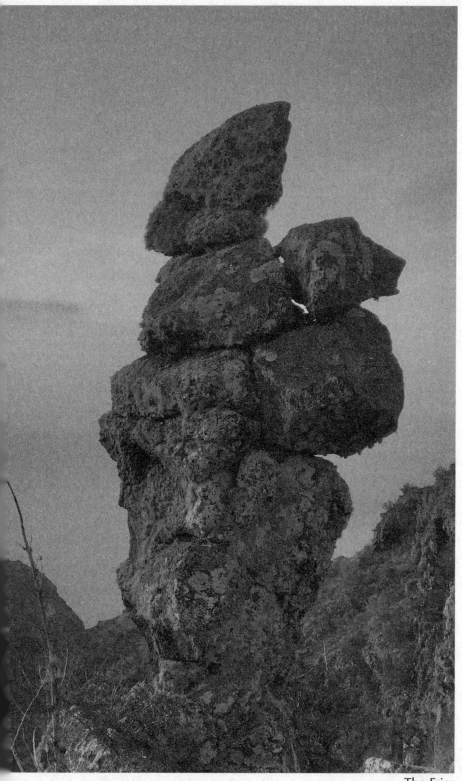

The Friar

'That's a terrified dog.'

A long empty silence followed. I cupped my hands to my face: 'ROSIEEEE... ROSIEEEE...' My echoing voice came back to mock me. 'The trouble is,' I sighed, 'if you shout a dog's name, they usually just listen. They tend not to answer.'

'Such a shame,' said Heather. 'She's been howling all morning.'

'She's tired, she's dehydrated, and to be honest, Heather, she's probably dying. Also, we don't know what injuries she has. There must be a reason she's trapped.' I turned to my steadfast colleague. 'Ken – fancy a hike?'

The route down Lemon Valley is a beautiful one, well maintained and delightfully scenic. But it takes no prisoners. Ken and I headed down the easy initial section, a pleasant, gently sloping country footpath shaded by trees before it turns into an ankle-breaking plummet of treacherous scree baked by the sweltering sun. After ten minutes or so we came to a natural viewpoint where the St Helena National Trust had thoughtfully placed a bench. We parked our rears and pricked our ears.

'This valley's vast, Ken. Rock faces, ledges, caverns and that thickly vegetated gut – she could be anywhere. No way can we search it.'

'No, Joe – it's hopeless. We've got more chance of setting sail in the *Papanui*.' That was the spatchcocked wreck of a burned-out steamship in James Bay.

'Yes!' It was worth a chuckle. 'Unless she talks to us. Come on, Rosie, shout for help.'

After a fruitless half hour, I suggested a different tactic. 'Ken, I know the way onto Friar's Ridge. We could listen from there.'

I navigated our climb up onto the ridge to gain a vantage-point. The Friar itself was about half a mile distant along the ridge towards the sea. Ken and I sat companionably on a finger of rock overhanging the chasm, chatting about work and scanning the opposite side of the gorge, where the road escaping Crack Plain made a tight switchback past the tiny church of St Martin's-in-the-Hills.

'You know, Joe,' mused Ken, deep in admiration of his own island, 'I've never been up here before. It certainly is a wonderful view.'

'You see! Not an entirely wasted afternoon.' I paused and patted him on the arm. 'OK, let's leave it for now. What I'll do, Ken, is come back here this evening after work and try again. Her hourglass is running out. Not long now and she'll be dead. But at least no one can say we haven't tried.'

True to my word, I returned that evening and sat on the National Trust bench with an uninspiring meal of Coke and crisps. Dusk drew in, and the scrubby vegetation all around started to vibrate with the staccato scritch of crickets broken by the occasional rustle of a foraging rodent. Small groups of fairy terns jinked high overhead, returning to their forest roosts after a hard day's fishing, their immaculate white plumage ablaze in the last rays of the setting sun. I tried shouting Rosie's name, then inanely, barking, as if dog to dog, but not one response came through the cooling air.

It was probably too late. Four whole days now without a drink. She could be asleep, but more likely slumped and moribund, possibly comatose, or of course finally released by her injuries. That single wail we'd heard had spoken volumes. It had been the wail of despair.

A fine rain began to patter down and intensify, seeping into both my mood and my jeans. It was time to abandon the quest.

Rain. Chilling, miserable rain.

AN IMPOSSIBLE CATCH

Day five dawned. That morning, Ken burst into the surgery where I was finishing a cat spay. He was excited, his face animated by hope rekindled. 'You won't believe it but... Rosie's started up again!'

'No way?' I paused my needle-holders. 'Tough girl. Right. This is it, Ken, our last and only chance.' I placed my final suture and threw down the instruments. 'Bring Rico too if he's available.'

Heather was waiting. 'She's weak now and it's harder to hear, but listen...' The four of us clung to the air, posed in frozen silence.

'There! There!' Rico whispered. Sure enough, a weak sobbing sound, pitiful, desperate and abandoned. But it was totally directionless.

I was running on adrenaline. 'Ken, the first thing you hit after Rosemary Plain is Friar's Ridge. She could of course have run through Crack Plain to the other side, but I'd take a punt on her being somewhere on this side. It halves the search area.' I waved my hand vaguely at the long wall of forbidding rock tapering off into the distance. 'I'll go back down the path and see if I can get a fix on her before she falls silent again. If she does though, I fear that'll be that.'

'OK, Joe. Rico and I will go up to St Martin's with the binos and scan the ridge from there, see if we can spot anything.'

'It's worth a try. But this landscape is extensive. She's going to be hard to find.' The whole rock face was pitted and scarred, every nook and cranny thrown into deep black shadow by the overhead sun: unhelpful camouflage for an equally black dog. And it ran for a mile and a half to the sea.

'Do you have your mobile?'

'Yes. But whether it'll work down there I have no idea.' Mobiles were a recent innovation for St Helena and her wild topography made coverage patchy, at best.

I half walked, half jogged along the Lemon Valley path, past the bench and then down a whole series of dug-out steps, descending rapidly from Friar's Ridge high above. Every now and then I paused, froze and strained my ears. Sometimes a minute or two passed, but Rosie kept it up, a soft wail subsiding into a whimper. I was gripped with determination. 'Keep it up, girl. Keep it up.' One good thing: it was definitely coming from the Friar's Ridge side of the gorge.

But there was something wrong. As the path continued to plummet, the sound became vaguer, more aloft and echoey, and yet still somewhere ahead. She was above me.

I examined the slope beneath the ridge with a critical eye: a series of broken mini escarpments laced with thickets and scrubby, stunted firs. It was littered with boulders, slabs and sharp-edged fragments of rock, cast off over millennia like flaking skin by the impressive wall of magma soaring above. I thought I could see a possible route and, leaving the security of the path, began to climb.

From stump to branch, rock to root, sometimes seeking a breach in a mini-escarpment where I could gain a few hand- and footholds to surmount the obstacle, I slowly wended my way up and still further along, guided by the occasional whimper. The sound remained doggedly ahead, and the valley floor was now becoming alarmingly distant, the path long since buried in its depths.

I had the wrong shoes, no rope and, it now occurred to me – rather late in the day – no veterinary equipment. My enthusiasm had led me into foolishness, and careful though I was, I began to appreciate that I could be creating my own crisis on top of the relatively minor matter of a lost dog. But I'm a vet. So long as I could hear the now very intermittent whimper, so long as Rosie called to me and I was on the trail, how could I possibly break off and give her up to a slow and wretched death?

But as I climbed, a new, rather distasteful realisation began to dominate my thoughts. The sheer rock face of Friar's Ridge was getting closer. If Rosie was anywhere on these sloping pediments, however tricky, she would have scrambled down. And with the unassailable wall of rock directly above, it could only mean one thing: she was lying at the base of the ridge, smashed and broken, perhaps paralysed with a fractured spine, and thanks to my failure to bring a kit, I had no means of humanely putting her to sleep. Which left one grisly alternative: bludgeoning her to death with a rock. Hardly the act of a skilled veterinary professional. I was not at all happy with myself.

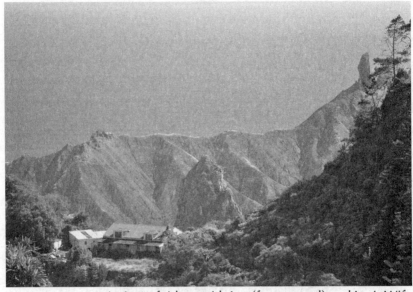

A view of ridges with Lot (foreground) and Lot's Wife
(on the farther ridge) from Mount Pleasant

When I finally reached the foot of the formidable rock face, I felt a buzz of excitement to see where I was. The valley seemed lost to me and, peering out from the scrub across the nothingness, I could just make out the white government Rover shimmering in the heat beneath the small, pale church of St Martin's, where, unbeknown to me, Rico and Ken had picked out my striped shirt with the binoculars and were monitoring my erratic progress.

There was a tiny sound, then silence, just the rattle of desiccated leaves in a light thermal breeze. Yet I could feel Rosie was close. She had to be, because the noises I had heard could never have been picked up at any great distance; but now all again was deathly quiet. Minutes passed and I began to fret. My senses were straining hard, heightened by adrenaline, the deeply hard-wired instincts of the hunter-gatherer scanning for the tiniest clue, the merest hint of an existence. Then thankfully she started again, short whimpers and whines, so low, so wavering and internalised, that they were barely audible. And they were still ahead of me.

A constant shower of debris down the rock face had created a narrow but welcome path along its base, and I moved swiftly along, bathed in wafts of heat radiating from the caramel-coloured magma. The whining continued but now, mysteriously, it seemed to be behind me. I stopped, hesitated, then backtracked. No, I was mistaken – it was ahead of me. I clasped my chin and looked up. It was above me. With some surprise I could see the foreshortened, stumpy figure of The Friar immediately overhead. I had come far. Beside me there was a secondary platform of rock, as if The Friar had a footstool, with a bare, unclimbable face. Rosie must be lying, broken, on top. I worked my way around the footstool to where it met the wall and found a chimney of jointed rock into which I could brace my limbs to haul myself up the ten or so feet and gain the top.

Not a whisker of a dog.

I sat wearily on the bald dome of the footstool, raised above the scrub with a magnificent vista stretching out beyond, perplexed by the ventriloquism of Rosie, now once again silent, and slightly perturbed by the thought that I had overcommitted and wouldn't be able to get down again. It is always easier to climb up than down, for which nature never saw fit to give us eyes in our toes.

I checked my mobile phone, but there was no signal. There was nothing to do but wait for Rosie to talk to me again. She had to know I was there.

'ROSIEEEE.... ROSIEEEE...!' It didn't work before, and it didn't work now. No response.

I stood up and a loose rock skittered away over the precipice. From the heavens above came a magnificent sound. A single bark. My eyes shot up.

'That's impossible.' Disbelief mingled with joy. 'Rosie! How in hell's name...'

High above, so perfectly in line with The Friar that it appeared to be below its buried feet, was a furry black head, pink tongue lolling and white teeth shining. Rosie had gone over the edge, and somehow lodged on a tiny concealed outcrop of rock. So concealed, in fact, that she appeared to project from the very rock face itself. Astonishing.

I quickly raised my hand. 'Stay, Rosie, stay!' I was suddenly worried that in her weakened state she would lose her footing, to plunge and smash at my feet, a ghastly prospect. 'Just stay. We're coming to get you.'

How could she be so alive after five days? Of course; it was that rain, the first rain in days, which I had so thoughtlessly cursed. Merciful, life-giving rain. Without a doubt it had given Rosie a vital drink, just enough to keep her bodily functions ticking over. As ever, I marvelled at the resilience of animals.

My excitement and sense of urgency gave me wings, and I had no trouble getting back down from The Friar's footstool. I looked across the valley to where the Rover was still parked beneath the distant church and cupped my hands around my mouth into my best foghorn. 'I'VE – FOUND – HER!'

The valley rumbled. 'WHAAAAAT?'

'I'VE – oh, forget it.' It was too far, and my yodelling days were over.

Further down I lost my tracks and had trouble descending past an escarpment. The mobile located a weak signal, and Rico picked up. 'Rico, I've found her. She's alive. It's quite incredible, but I'll tell you later. At the moment though I can't find the path. Where is it?'

Rico gave a small laugh. 'It's OK, I've been watching you. Go on to the left. More... more... a little more. That's it. Now it's just below you.'

At the top of the path Ken and Rico were waiting for me in the vehicle, with huge expectant grins on their questioning faces. I was soaked in sweat and blowing like a horse at the end of a hard gallop. But I didn't care. I was feeling triumphant.

'Well,' said Ken. 'Spill the beans. What's the story?'

'Well, guys, the long and the short of it is... we need the fire brigade.'

SEND FOR THE CAVALRY

'Alan, we've got a good one for you.' Ken relayed the details down the phone.

Alan 'Mackerel', fire brigade chief, sounded a little shocked. 'She's where?'

'As it happens,' Ken continued, 'Joe knows a route and can lead you there.'

We agreed to convene outside the Guinea Grass Community Centre on the other side of Friar's Ridge. When I arrived, I was immediately impressed by their massive presence: two fire engines and a stretch Rover in a blaze of red and St Helena crests, and an army of blue-uniformed firemen hauling out and checking equipment.

Alan, ever jovial, greeted me with a handshake and a flash of teeth. The others gathered round. 'Are you sure? It doesn't sound possible.'

'Close to impossible, but she's there all right. Have any of you ever been up to The Friar?'

Heads shook with murmurs of no. 'As a child,' said Jason, 'but never since.'

'Well, it'll be a good training exercise,' added Alan. 'We'll take a team of eight. Gear up, guys.'

I led the string of eight firemen with their backpacks and coils of climbing rope, their carabiners clanking from their harnesses, along my tortuous route to The Friar. Their orange climbing helmets bobbed along the ridge and were seen for miles around. After half an hour we came out onto the small platform, my spectacular picnic site. The Friar looked down benevolently on a gathering the likes of which it had never seen before. The team gazed back up at its towering hulk with a mixture of awe and wonder.

'Impressive. So much larger than you expect.' Alan was staring at the loose stack of boulders that formed The Friar's head and cowl. 'But I don't think we'll rope around it. Looks like it would topple over and kill us all.'

I was craning my neck over the precipice. 'I can't see Rosie, Alan, but she's there somewhere.' A wave of disappointment swept over me. 'Oh, shit... unless she's fallen.'

Alan, ever calm, gave a philosophical shrug. 'We'll soon know.'

The team began to rig up the equipment, looking for alternative places to secure and belay the ropes. Jason could see a small, loose chute of rock going over the edge beside The Friar and got tempted. He spreadeagled his body and inched himself confidently over the rim of hanging debris. He was an experienced climber and used to collecting goat fodder from precipitous locations.

'There's no dog here...' he began. But the rock was foul, what climbers call choss, and there was a swish and clatter of falling stones as he dropped from sight.

'Jason!' shouted one of his colleagues in alarm. My heart pounded. Heaven forbid that I would be the cause of sending a fireman to his cherry-jam death for the sake of one lost dog. I felt sickened to the bones and could barely look. But an orange helmet popped above the rim.

'It's OK,' said Jason merrily, oblivious of our concern and waving a bloodied finger in the air. 'Just my hand.'

'Rope, Jason.' Alan scowled.

Once secured, Jason's colleagues belayed him down the rock face. The tension was palpable. In my mind I was now convinced Rosie had tried to follow me when I had set off back down the path and had become a crumpled bag of shattered bones marking the spot where I had stood just two hours before.

Still further Jason was lowered. 'No – she's not here.' I was overwhelmed by intense disappointment.

He disappeared over a bulge in the rock face and the cry that we had all been waiting for echoed across the gorge.

'I CAN SEE HER!'

It was almost beyond belief. Running cross-country in her blind panic she had met with Friar's Ridge, hit the oblique rock contours leading up to the saddle on which The Friar stood, gone over the edge, and then slipped and fallen some thirty feet or so, no doubt scrabbling desperately at the rock face to save her own life.

And then the miracle. She had struck a small balcony of rock, the only barrier between her and certain death.

Alan sent down another fireman and they worked away out of sight below the bulge in the rock face. Rosie was friendly, but the logistics of securing a dog in a harness designed for a human are distinctly tricky. Some time passed before she was suitably cocooned in a spider's web of strapping, and we were confident enough to haul her up the rock face. But, at last, haul her we did.

Rosie stood beside The Friar, wagging her tail and staring down at what might have been, happy to be back in the company of humans. I pulled a lead from around my waist and quickly clipped it onto her collar. She was mine now. I patted her and stroked her head. 'Well done, girl. Well done.'

There was a general air of merriment and well-deserved congratulations for a job well done with the best of possible outcomes. Meanwhile, I checked her over. Her long-haired coat was lank and she was marginally dehydrated, but all in all she was in remarkably good shape. A fireman pulled a bottle of water from his backpack and glugged its contents into his upturned helmet. All watched with immense satisfaction and nods of approval as she noisily lapped it up, drools of stringy saliva hanging from her parched lips. I partly walked but mostly carried her back to the fire vehicles and after an exuberant debriefing, took her to the surgery for overnight food and water, discharging her the next day.

THE BEEKEEPER

It was the time of COVID-19, and the pandemic was at its height.

St Helena had remained COVID free by virtue of her isolation – for once, not a tyranny but a blessing – and one of my roles was as Proper Officer, an archaic title embedded in the superbly named Formidable Diseases Regulations. I and my fellow officers, backed by a full team from Public Health, stood in a row behind two-metre distanced tables, shuffling forms as passengers, all anonymised by masks, came through from one of the occasional relief flights at the new airport to be briefed and have the fear of god put into them. But nicely.

A public health assistant placed the next form on my table, and I scanned through the pages then glanced up. Tony Leo stood before me.

'Tony! I'm so glad to see you back. You look good.'

'Getting there, Joe, getting there.' A fit man with a healthy lifestyle, much of it spent nurturing his bees, he'd nonetheless had a triple bypass operation to reinvigorate his oxygen-starved heart. And he genuinely looked chipper and rosy cheeked. 'The chest still aches a bit, but that'll pass. Joe,' he went on, 'thank you for all you've done with Rosie.'

'Oh... that's my huge pleasure, Tony.' A beloved family pet is so integral to supporting a recuperating owner.

I then went on to fulfil my task, bellowing instructions to overcome the muffle of the mask and the two-metre gap, and threatening Tony with up to six months imprisonment and a £5,000 fine for any breach of quarantine; yet in cushioned and friendly terms. St Helena has a dangerously susceptible population and only a cottage hospital to cope, so the penalties were some of the severest in the world. How medieval COVID had made us: lotions, potions, masks and retribution.

Tony Leo was reunited with Rosie and rapidly returned to his former good health. A win–win.

THE BARD'S CURE

Ten months later, I was at my desk working through emails when the phone rang. It was the Governor's personal assistant, Linda.

'The Governor would like you to attend a ceremony at Plantation on Wednesday the sixth of October. Can you come?'

'A ceremony? Yes, delighted.' The kitchens of Plantation House had something of a reputation and always turned out generous platters of tasty finger food combining the finest of local ingredients; and no doubt there would be a glass or two of Foreign Office-financed hospitality wine to wash the food down. Apart from that, I always delighted in soaking up the rich Georgian heritage of Plantation House: the scent of waxed hardwood floors; the glint of burnished East India Company silverware; the glitter of crystal chandeliers; and the tall, dadoed walls of foxed lithographs and oil paintings, each picture with its own tale to tell.

It soon transpired that Rico and Ken were also invited, and when we mounted the steps of Plantation House's voluminous porch and rubbed shoulders with Alan, Jason and the rest of the fire crew, the penny dropped. We mingled in the Blue Room with its padded armchairs and chaises longues, sipping our glasses of wine and beer and savouring the delicacies floated around by Plantation House's unerringly neat and efficient staff. Dr Philip Rushbrook, Governor of St Helena, Ascension and

Tristan da Cunha – surely a portfolio with a greater ratio of sea to land than any other – held the floor. Slight, grey haired and bespectacled, he spoke, as ever, with quick wit and piercing logic. He was my fourth governor.

'We're gathered here today to celebrate a somewhat unusual event. The rescue of a dog.' He went on to call us up one by one, present an envelope, and shake our hands for a photocall.

Inside the envelope was a crisp, crested certificate printed on dimpled cartridge paper which read:

CERTIFICATE FOR AN ACT OF BRAVERY
awarded to
DR JONATHAN DOUGLAS HOLLINS
in recognition of bravery in extraordinary circumstances.
CITATION
For performing an act of bravery on 5 January 2021
by being instrumental in the difficult rescue of a dog
whose life was in peril after falling on to a cliff ledge.
P. Rushbrook
Governor

It was a great honour. I was asked to recount the tale, which I did, congratulating the fire brigade on their immediacy, professionalism and compassion, and not least – to many laughs – on sacrificing a fireman's helmet to dog saliva. But the simple truth was that I delighted in the challenge, loved the hike and had a fantastically rewarding goal to achieve: to save a little life and return a beloved pet to a man whom I liked and admired and who had just had a major heart operation. And anyway, bravery is but a wafer away from recklessness.

Furthermore, it was all down to Rosie.

As the Bard so accurately says, blind fear had given way to reason, and having found safer footing and fearing the worst, Rosie found the cure; she had called for help and drawn us in to an almost unfindable location. And is there anything so nakedly honest as that primal cry from a stricken animal?

It wasn't me who had provided the solution to Rosie's problem. It was Rosie.

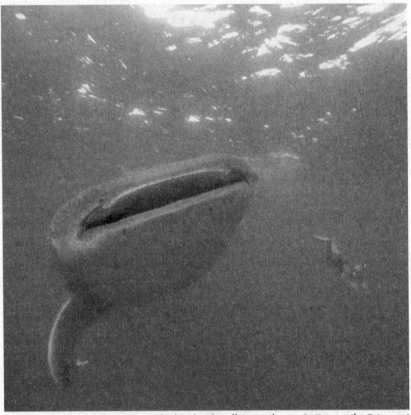

Me freediving with a whale shark off St Helena © Dr Attila Frigyesi

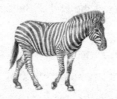

HORSES AND ZEBRAS

For when the One Great Scorer comes
To mark against your name
He writes not that you won or lost
But how you played the game

Grantland Price, 'Alumnus Football' (1908)
A framed quote on my brother's bedside table,
moral guidance from our grandfather.

BIZARRE BEZOARS

'Don't look for zebras when there are only horses' goes one of the principal axioms of medical diagnosis trotted out at college. In other words, common things happen commonly.

Sure they do, but Professor Jennings, one of my learned tutors, who had written the authoritative tome on animal pathology and for whom I had the profoundest respect, pointed out the slight flaw in the axiom.

'It's incomplete,' he advised. 'Dangerously misleading. If you only look for horses, you'll never find the zebras. And they are there in their very many forms.'

Less zebras perhaps, more chimeras, but yes, rare conditions are only rare individually. In their entirety, they are common and occur frequently, though you might come across each one just once in a professional career. Thanks to this sound advice, when symptoms and findings don't add up, I have always tried to hunt down the elusive zebra. And I knew, as I post-mortemed the kid goat and laid my hands on what felt like a fleet of bobbing corks in its rumen, that I was onto a zebra of a most peculiar stripe.

I slit open the wall of the rumen, and a cascade of buoyant khaki-coloured felt marbles flowed out on a stream of pungent, grassy fluid. Astonishing. I had only ever seen these in a museum.

Bezoars.

The case was an enigma from the start. When I had first examined the kid goat – then just barely alive – at Mount Pleasant, it presented with all the symptoms of grass sickness. Dilated pupils, a paralysed bowel and stone-like faeces called faecoliths. The only problem with this diagnosis was that grass sickness, or equine dysautonomia, a fatal disruption of the autonomic nervous system, is an obscure toxicosis of horses found in very specific locations. (Years ago, just after I qualified, it was also mysteriously imitated by a flurry of cases in cats; called Key-Gaskell syndrome or feline dysautonomia, it disappeared as rapidly as it appeared and was suspected to be caused by an unintended toxic ingredient of some proprietary cat food.)

But caprine dysautonomia? If so, it would be an index case, the first ever recorded. That would be a zebra and a half. In both the cat and the horse, it is some form of toxin at play. Did I have a weird, one-off poisoning here? And how could I explain the curious presence of bezoars? An intriguingly knotty problem to solve.

The word bezoar is derived from the Persian *padzahr*, meaning 'antidote'. Bezoars were highly prized and considered to be endowed with powerful properties, often worn around the neck as talismans, guarding particularly – and ironically as it turned out in this case – against poisonings. Queen Elizabeth I had one embedded in a bejewelled finger ring.

The majority are trichobezoars made of hair, the most extreme version of which, Rapunzel syndrome, is found mainly in girls who chew their manes and involves a large gastric bezoar with a ponytail trailing into the small intestine – though with not a prince in sight. Phytobezoars, made of plant material, are considered unusual and are largely associated with poor gut motility. Which was interesting, as that was exactly what I had diagnosed, and these bezoars were definitely of plant material.

It happens that Mount Pleasant, a historic dwelling with Napoleonic and East India Company connections up on a high, picturesque ridge, is owned by a respected biologist and conservationist, Rebecca Cairns-Wicks, along with her husband Greg. Becky rolled a bezoar analytically between her fingers and suddenly raised her head with a jerk of recognition.

'I know what this is! Follow me.'

We returned to the scene of the crime, the goat paddock, where an extensive overgrowth of vegetation hung over the banks. Dense thickets of aggressively invasive wild ginger mingled with lanky bushes dangling pendulous white flowers the size of ice cream cones.

'The yellow ginger lily, *Hedychium flavescens*. The underside of each leaf has an indumentum, a covering of fine siliceous hairs called trichomes, and the goats browse it. Look.' She plucked a leaf and rubbed away the felty coating. It balled between her fingertips. 'There's your bezoar,' she announced triumphantly.

'And what's this?' The ginger showed signs of cropping, but so too did the lower limbs of the lanky bushes, which were heady with a suffocating bordello scent.

'Here we call it Ladies' Petticoats. It's Angels' Trumpets, *Brugmansia suaveolens*, one of the datura family. Poisonous, of course.'

Aha.

And so it is, rich in the paralytics of the autonomic nervous system, scopolamine, hyoscyamine and atropine, all closely related to curare as used by indigenous Amazonians on their arrow heads to immobilise their prey. Or a kid goat with experimental tastes in foliage. So I wasn't being fanciful after all. It was indeed a one-off case like grass sickness; the kid was paralysing his gut with datura, then fuelling the bezoars with ginger, the cohesive siliceous hairs slowly building up in the rumen like a snowball rolling down a hill. It was the neatest accidental collaboration between two intermingled plants that I had ever seen or could ever have conceived of.

I had my source material. I had my paralytic. And now I had cornered, trapped and boxed my zebra.

The kid billy goat had a twin, a female, and since siblings invariably copy each other, we caught her up and I probed my fingertips deep into her abdomen. She seemed well. But...

'I don't believe it, Becky. I have never felt this before. She's packed with bezoars. And they're big.' High on the right flank, so tame and relaxed was this young nanny, I could grasp several large bezoars floating within the roof of her rumen.

Becky was equally fascinated. 'Well, she's not for breeding. These two goats are the product of a mismating, so when she's up to weight we're going to slaughter her. You're welcome to come along and see what we find.'

Several months later by the outbuildings of Mount Pleasant, I was examining a row of furry dice, much larger than her sibling's, intriguingly shaped into cuboids by the tight confines of the rumen. I have my souvenir bezoar beside me now, felted, featherweight, and still aromatically redolent of goat, my personal antidote against all evils and cure for all ills. That'd be something – the vet's equivalent of a magic wand.

If only.

But perhaps in an odd, roundabout way the bezoars did bring good fortune to my door, in the shape of a monster of a project.

Over the following months the Ladies' Petticoats and the yellow ginger lily, for all their ornamental charm, were shown no mercy, and Becky set about eliminating them. As it was, she and Greg had poured their resources into clearing the dense swathes of invasives that choked and smothered their pastures, replacing them with vulnerable St Helena endemics and restoring the landscape to something resembling its former glory. She didn't need the bezoars to drive her; the endemics were almost her *raison d'être*.

While revisiting Mount Pleasant and admiring her efforts, Becky grabbed my elbow and pulled me onto a path. 'Come and have a proper look.'

She walked me up a steep fist of rock to an old military lookout, the Mount. At 650 metres it commands a view some sixty miles out to sea and takes in the whole, grippingly wild landscape of St Helena's fiercest side: the phonolite volcanic plug of Lot, protruding like a plump baguette; the hunched and scowling Lot's Wife on a distant ridge; the tumbled nursery of Lot's Children lying between the two; the self-explanatory Gates of Chaos and Devil's Garden; the black columnar Asses Ears; the spookily realistic Gorilla's Head; and the petrified sails of the Man O' War. These outcrops are formed from the gutted interior of the primary volcano, tortured and tumultuous and with names to match. Becky pointed down into the dense jungle of trees and thickets on the other side of the Mount where two gables thrust their tall, cocoa-stone chimneys up through the branches, cloaked in parasitic saplings.

'That's Rose Cottage,' she explained. 'A complete ruin. Destroyed by the white ant.' The wood termite, introduced to St Helena by a Brazilian slave ship, caused the collapse of many buildings in Jamestown, hence the prevalence of steel

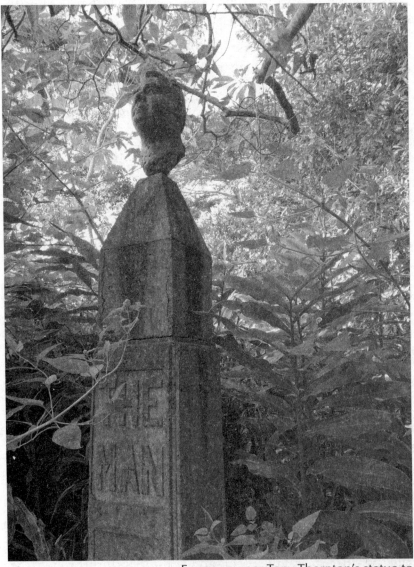

Former owner Tony Thornton's statue to himself in the grounds of Rose Cottage

railway-track roof beams and the magnificent cast-iron staircase in the Castle. 'It was a Georgian mansion built in about 1820 by the son-in-law of Sir William Doveton, the Secretary of the East India Company. More recently it was owned by Tony Thornton, a dynamic businessman who split island opinion with his projects. The government felt threatened by him, so they banished him overseas sometime in the 1970s. He's dead now and nobody really knows who owns it. Do you want to see his statue?'

'Statue?'

We fought our way through the vegetation and fallen boughs, swinging a machete to clear a path. The ruins were extensive: a deep basement filled with the rubble of collapsed walls; living room fireplaces suspended on lime-mortared chimney breasts, their brass tracery intact and verdigrised; and a dark, dank coffee and banana plantation throttled by invasives all screaming for the light. We came, quite surreally, to a tall monolith of concrete bearing a well-sculpted bronze head: Tony Thornton. Erected by him before his death, the bust gazed out like a Caesar from the brink of a precipice across what should have been a phenomenal view, now throttled and obscured by vegetation. Bold, raised capitals cast in the concrete proclaimed: 'THE MAN'.

I would never have had the nerve, let alone the ego. He must have been interesting.

At the base lay a wreath of bright plastic flowers. I picked it up. 'From all at Solomons,' the label read. Solomons is a company he virtually came to own before he was kicked out and it was nationalised.

Rose Cottage sunk her talons into me. I was gripped. Here was a ridiculous project. I had to have it, and I had just unwittingly picked up the key to the lock.

I contacted Mandy Peters, the warm and cheerful current CEO of Solomons, and asked her what she knew. 'Yes,' she confirmed. 'We laid that wreath when Tony died. His ashes are there. If you like I can give you an email address for one of his daughters.'

I did like, and before long I was in touch with all five of Thornton's offspring, now scattered around the world. I put together a package, citing local house prices and the state of the site, made a fair offer, and they accepted. No going back. The solicitors unravelled the legal maze of a lost trust, and I found myself owner of a colossal, alluringly beautiful, money-gobbling, three-and-a-half acre retirement project; inaccessibly remote, buried in jungle, and teetering on a rain-soaked, wind-swept precipice. A piece, in fact, of St Helena's precious cloud forest on the central spine of the island.

And with it, a plantation of overgrown green-tipped Bourbon Arabica coffee trees. My very own coffee.

What's not to like?

Clearly, though, I had taken complete leave of my senses.

CARDBOARD LAMBS

It isn't every day you dig up a foo dog.

I had been dedicating months of evenings and weekends to clearing the long, steep track up to Rose Cottage, choked with gorse, ginger, aloe, flax and fallen timber. It was gruelling work. After felling a few trees and digging up their bumpy roots, I finally had access for my twenty-five-year-old Land Rover Defender, and no longer had to hump my tools up from Greg's driveway way below.

Teeny visited on mercy missions clutching reviving bars of chocolate, the occasional sandwich and an evening cider or two, always accompanied by Che, the softest, loopiest, most devoted springer spaniel you could hope to find. A dog reads the world through its nose, so acutely can it detect the myriad molecular residues of nature's comings and goings. It was sheer unalloyed pleasure to watch Che work the ground for rats, or to hear him come crashing through the tangled undergrowth to seek me out. I did, though, corral off a wild bees' nest established in a pile of masonry, as his klutz-like zigzagging would have soon led him into a whole buzz of hot water.

I was sitting on the Rover's tailgate one afternoon rehydrating with a cup of Thermos tea having just hacked through to the old stables. They had been flattened by the rotting trunk of a fallen colossus. The whole structure was so submerged in jungle that I felt like Hiram Bingham rediscovering Machu Picchu. The stable block had clearly been built by frustrated masons of high ambition. Protruding from the soil next to a Pisa-like tower of unnecessarily massive quoins, I had spotted

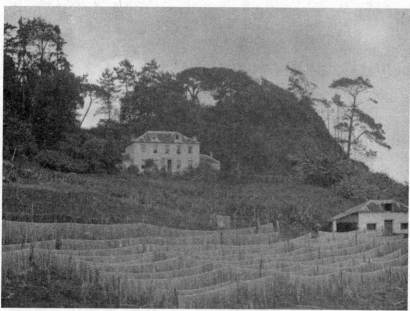

Rose Cottage and her flax farm in the nineteenth century

a large, biscuity section of glazed pot with some sort of decorative handle. I yanked it out, and the handle glared back at me angrily. It was a Chinese foo dog.

I washed it off and admired its features while I slurped at my tea: bulging eyes, face of a Pekingese, lion-cub ears, ferocious snarl, all coated in the remnants of a yellow-green celadon glaze with hints of gilding. A classic East India Company import.

This was superbly propitious. Foo dogs or imperial guardian lions were traditionally erected in pairs to protect property and ward off unwanted visitors. It was an unlikely prospect, but how I would love to unearth its partner. Then I could mount them on the gate jambs to send a tongue-in-cheek message to all and sundry.

I drained my tea and considered the strange sensation in my throat when I swallowed. I'd woken a few days before to the feeling of a small lump, like a lodged bolus of food. But I dismissed it as trivial.

The dreaded vibration in my pocket warned me that the emergency mobile was about to trill.

Theoretically I had retired several months before, but in reality, I had been inveigled into providing cover in the absence of a suitable replacement, and anyway felt morally and ethically obliged to provide essential services. I could hardly sit back and watch animals die.

It was Chopsie.

'What's up, Chops?' Clayton Andrews was an invaluable, long-serving member of the veterinary team, and I had a lot of time for him. As a child he had undergone years of treatment for leukaemia, finally conquering it, and had therefore endured more suffering, both physical and mental, than anyone should at that age. His body was pocked with scars from the repeated insertion of medical implements. He had missed out on a lot of schooling, but along with a doting family, his experiences had somehow made him extremely well-grounded, impeccably honest, serene and helpful. He was also a very competent livestock owner, his particular forte being sheep and goat husbandry.

'Sorry to disturb you on your long holiday.' A slight chortle at my expense. 'Thought you'd like some work. Steve Biggs has been losing lambs. He's got another one down and he'd like you to take a look.'

'Oh, I didn't know. Is it the Barber's Pole?' This fiendish thread of a worm with a drill bit for a mouth was a scourge of the island's sheep and goats. It lives in the 'true' stomach, the abomasum, tapping into the blood supply as if drilling for oil, draining off their essence. The red spiral of blood in its intestine gives it the layman's name, reminiscent of the traditional pole above a barber's shop doorway. Its true name is *Haemonchus contortus* – my murderous, multitudinous, implacable enemy, a gift from Africa courtesy of the EIC.

'Don't think so. The lambs aren't pale. But something's badly wrong with them. They just don't flow right.'

Chopsie's canny herdsman's instincts were evidently being tweaked. 'OK, sure, I'll call round this evening after I've finished up here. At least I can get a decent brew of coffee.'

Steve and Maureen of Farm Lodge were their usual genial selves. 'Follow me,' said Steve breathlessly, weaving between his plethora of sheds and vehicles and clambering over a fence into the sheep paddocks with Katy Dog in tow. Steve had subdivided his large paddock into thirteen smaller ones to adopt the system of 'mob grazing'. It's a good plan designed to draw the maximum yield from the pasture, to graze and move before the sward is cropped to the ground, leaving more blade to photosynthesise and speeding regrowth. 'Sorry to bother you. I know you're semi-retired, but it's now seven or eight lambs out of the twenty, and they all seem to go the same way. They lose the use of their hindquarters.'

'No, it's fine, Steve. That's far too many and there has to be an answer.'

We ducked into a small wooden hut where a six-month-old lamb lay prostrate on a bed of straw while Shaun, Steve's helper, was encouraging it to drink. It appeared to be in good condition, as were all of Steve's sheep, amply fed not just with grass but bundles of cut fodder and buckets of sheep cube.

It was a straightforward diagnosis. I performed a full neurological examination and checked the lamb's vitals. Front half: perfectly alert and responsive. Rear half: paralysed. The lamb was paraplegic. There was evidence of upper motor neurone degeneration, of a destruction within the spinal cord.

I walked through the flock. The adult ewes were in fine condition, fat even. The lambs, now weaned and in their own set of paddocks, were varied, and one had a bunny-hopping gait.

'And the symptoms have been the same for all the lambs you've lost?'

'Yes. After they go off their hind legs, they go on feeding for a week or so, then usually start to deteriorate and either die or we call in your team to have them put down.'

'Steve, this is classic late-onset copper deficiency of fast-growing lambs,' I surmised with absolute conviction. 'Swayback. And that bunny-hopping lamb there looks as if it's next.'

'But why have all the ram lambs been affected first?' put in Shaun.

'That's interesting. Probably because they grow the fastest. They have the greater need.'

It all made perfect sense. I explained how copper deficiency was quite prevalent on the island – leached volcanic soils, competition with iron and sulphur – and that, among its many other roles, copper was critical in the development of the spinal cord. If lambs are damaged *in utero* and born with swayback, it is generally too late to correct the damage, but if they develop it as they grow, the deficiency can be compensated for and the damage at least halted in its tracks. The pathology involved a loss of myelin along the spinal nerve tracts, the vital insulating material that allows nerves to conduct in the same way as an electric cable. 'I'll get the team to come round and inject them all with copper,' I added in conclusion.

Copper is a fickle element: some species thrive on it, such as pigs, others are more sensitive to its toxicity, like sheep. But we all need it. I will never forget, as a student, visiting a farm in the Lake District to assist with post-mortems where the farmer, standing over us with a look of despair and red-rimmed eyes, had unwittingly killed all his pedigree rams by feeding them leftover pig food.

As Hippocrates would have it: first, do no harm. We would cautiously inject only a moderate dose.

A close second rule, in my opinion, is to take a very thorough history. Oh Hollins, Hollins, Hollins. In my haste and certainty, and keenness to get back to jungle bashing at Rose Cottage, I had failed to follow my own rule.

A huge zebra was lurking in the shadows.

It wasn't long before Steve was on the phone again. 'I'm sorry, Joe. Maybe it was too late, but we've got another one. And it's not the bunny-hopper.'

I was soon back in the hut, testing reflexes and checking vital signs. 'Well, it's the same. Paraplegic. But I'm surprised I didn't spot this lamb a couple of weeks ago. It must have been coming on.'

'No, no, you wouldn't have,' piped up Shaun. 'That's the whole point. The lamb was perfectly normal until I went into the paddock with the feed. They all came galloping down, then this one suddenly hit the deck and started dragging its legs.'

'What?' I almost barked. There it was, the crucial fact I had failed to ascertain.

'Yes. They've all been the same. It happens suddenly.'

I froze, trance-like, over the recumbent lamb, my head spinning with physiology, my analysis plunging down a funnel of limited possibilities, rapidly eliminating the differentials to come to one inescapable conclusion.

'Oh my god. I know what this is. Impossible.' No – it was possible. 'I've only ever seen this once before, Steve, in...' and I had to laugh, but in disbelief, '...in Burmese kittens.' The kittens were being reared by a breeder who thought she knew best and was just feeding them raw meat, virtually devoid of the calcium needed for growing bones. 'I've been an idiot. Wrong mineral. I'm sorry, this isn't copper deficiency at all.'

'Kittens? I hate to point out the obvious and say these aren't kittens, but, well, these aren't kittens.' Steve was staring at me with commendable restraint. 'Go on then. What do you think it is this time?'

'Forget the kittens for a minute. It's nutritional secondary hyperparathyroidism. It has to be.'

Steve pulled a wry smile and shook his magnificent white mane. 'No, none the wiser.'

'It's logical, Steve. This is a sudden onset paralysis, not a slow one, and it's caused by exercise. If it were a single lamb, you'd say, "What bad luck, the lamb's slipped a disc or had an embolism." But it's not bad luck. You've had eight of them.'

'Still none the wiser.'

'Bear with me. It's calcium deficiency. But not of your standard sort.'

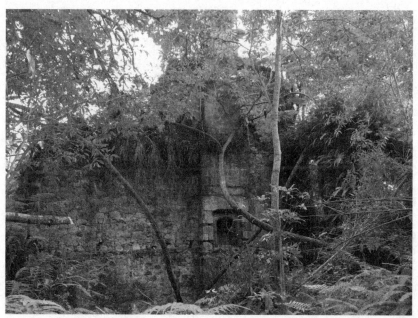

Rose Cottage as she is now

'What's the standard sort?'

'You know, you have a ewe heavy in lamb, she goes floppy, I give her a calcium injection and she gets up and walks away. You've had one, remember?'

'Oh yes. Mint Sauce. Poor old girl.'

'So... calcium is vital for many functions: nerve conduction, muscle contraction and so on. If blood levels fall too low, we mammals die. To avoid this, evolution gave us a gland called the parathyroid right here in the neck just to maintain blood calcium levels.' I prodded my voicebox. 'Lambs are making skeletons, so they have a high demand for calcium, but the gland quarries calcium from the bones if the blood levels drop dangerously low. After all, what's more important, strong bones or dropping dead? However, the gland functions on the basis that this is just a temporary solution to the problem. Too much quarrying, and the bones turn to cardboard. Wet cardboard. They don't even fracture. They buckle and fold.' I reached the grisly and inevitable conclusion. 'These lambs are breaking their own backs.'

He groaned. 'Not good. Not good at all. But what have we done wrong?'

'Nothing, Steve. You feed your sheep well. Just look at your ewes, they're a bit obese if anything. It'll be a conspiracy of factors. You're mob grazing with faster grass recovery and it's been a very warm, wet year, which means lush grass of poor nutritional value. These are acidic volcanic soils, famously poor for calcium. And there is bound to be another factor, a competing mineral like phosphate, or too little magnesium.'

'Right. So, how do we stop it? We can't afford to lose any more.'

'First I have to prove it. I'll draw some bloods and take them to the hospital lab. And I'm afraid I want that lamb. We'll put it to sleep, then I'll X-ray the body and do a post-mortem. Meanwhile, Steve, treat the rest as if they're made of glass. No more running about. Confine them. Otherwise they'll snap.'

Steve groaned, shook his mane once more, then offered the only possible comfort in that grim scenario. 'Coffee?'

Back at Agriculture, I laid the euthanised lamb out on the lead-lined table and collimated the light beam of the X-ray generator along the lumbar spine. Kerry Sim pushed the digital cassette underneath and I took a couple of shots. Kerry was my irreplaceable treasure, both a practice manager and a para-veterinarian. She overflowed with initiative and, like the best veterinary assistants, was almost clairvoyant of my needs when assisting with surgical procedures.

We had a useful collaboration with the hospital in town, using their digital developer, although it did mean a delay before I could analyse the plates. The evidence should be on the X-ray, but first I would do a very simple if crude and brutal test.

Kerry set out the post-mortem instruments and I made a single incision parallel to the spine, then dissected a window through the muscle to reach the thickest and hardest part of the vertebral bone, the vertebral body. She handed me a two-inch, heavy gauge needle. It slid through the bone as if it were clay.

I handed the needle to Kerry. 'Kerry, feel this.'

She thrust in the needle and her eyes nearly popped out of her head. 'That's terrible. There's no resistance.'

'Wait until you see the X-rays.'

The X-rays were even more startling. At first, I could barely discern the spine at all, just its ghostly outline. The density was little different from that of the surrounding soft tissue. But the wonder of digital radiography is that it's manipulable. Gone are the days of wet developing under a red light and discarding your failures. I played with the exposure, even reversed the contrast, a neat trick to enhance definition, and a faint spinal column appeared. The last two lumbar vertebrae, the point of thrust against the pelvis, had crumpled together like a wet, discarded dishcloth. When the blood results came back, the calcium levels, which the parathyroid gland should still have been maintaining at the expense of the skeleton, were lethally low. QED.

A ZEBRA COMES HOME

Meanwhile, the strange lump in my throat had persisted and since it had by now progressed to an unpleasant strangulating sensation, I booked an appointment with the proficient Dr Kamar. She performed a thorough examination, could neither feel or see any interfering mass, and arranged for a precautionary CT scan.

While I waited for the scan, I took my health concerns to the best place I could think of: the sea. Not only my personal health: we had no calcium supplements on the island such as shell grit to solve Steve and Maureen's problem – and I'd had an idea. It was a balmy tropical evening, and the covey of boats in James Bay wallowed placidly on their moorings. I pulled on my shorty wetsuit, fins, mask and snorkel, and threw myself off the Middle Steps into the lucent waters.

The sea surrounding St Helena is, to me, the island's great glory. It has never been heavily fished, never been trashed by trawl nets or shellfish dredges, and is thus blessed with the whole spectrum of oceanic life. The shoals of fish, especially the confetti clouds of the endemic cunning fish, are so abundant and healthy that they often obscure the view. The sharks are out there but warded off by our guardians and their arch enemies, roaming pods of pantropical dolphins.

For the diver, the Bay never disappoints. It is littered with an astonishing number of cannon and anchors, amorphous iron debris, and the carcasses of ships, chief among them the SS *Papanui*, a 130-metre-long steamship lying in twelve metres of water inside the moorings. She had burned to the waterline in 1911, all 472 passengers and crew safely evacuated, and now provided the island with her best artificial reef, blossoming with life. I duckdived around her rudder, where her stout sternpost still projects above the surface, swimming through nonchalant shoals of rainbow runners, goat fish, trumpet fish and albacore tuna, and ran my fingers through the gritty sand around her redundant stern anchor to check its quality. No – it wouldn't do.

She wasn't the only wreck in range. Despite her remote location, St Helena has experienced war. On the other side of the moorings lies a more tragic hulk, the RFA *Darkdale*, our deep dive site in forty metres of water, and an official war grave. In 1941, Kapitan Karl-Friedrich Merten of U-boat U-68 slammed an extravagant four torpedoes into her, tearing her in two with the loss of forty-one souls. Only 300 metres away lie the rusting cannon and piles of tin ingots from a more ancient lady, the Dutch East Indiaman man o' war, the *Witte Leeuw* or *White Lion*, which in 1613 scrapped with the Portuguese and promptly exploded, blowing her crew, timbers, peppercorns, porcelain and 1,311 diamonds to kingdom come. The diamonds, we are told, have never been found. Hmm – I wonder...

Although a diamond or two wouldn't go amiss, I was after a more mundane form of carbon: seashells, or calcium carbonate.

Back on the wharf I watched an islander raking barnacles off the keel of a fishing boat and scooped up a handful. Unfortunately, they were not only contaminated by the rotting flesh of these little crustaceans but also toxic flakes of anti-fouling paint. Again, they wouldn't do.

My other distractions had blurred my lateral thinking. The solution was already in my head, and I had used it ten years before to strengthen the eggshells of our hens in the government poultry unit.

Of course: Darwin's aeolian sands.

St Helena is not gifted with white sandy beaches. Her steep shores and high flanks commit shell debris to the deep, hence my snorkelling gambit. But it wasn't always so. In another age, when sea levels were lower and the coastline gentler, white coralline beaches abounded, and the strong prevailing south-east trades on the windward side of the island would 'winnow' and 'drift' the finer particles of 'calcareous dust' – as Darwin put it – into the becalming lacunae of the higher valleys. These sands had been quarried extensively by the military for kilning into lime mortar to build the girdle of defences that plugged every flaw in the island's already forbidding coastline.

When I first came to the island, I had used several pints of malt vinegar from my larder to dissolve samples of this sand, proving that it was 75 per cent calcium carbonate. I should have read Darwin and saved the vinegar for my tuna and chips. He put it at 70 per cent. Who am I to quibble with the great man over 5 per cent?

'Steve, I have a plan.' I was hovering over Steve's water trough in the lamb paddocks waving a pH strip in his face like a bottle of smelling salts. I was excited because it was all coming together. 'Look at this. A pH of five. Your water is incredibly acidic.'

'Almost good for pickling my shallots. So how does this help?'

'I'm going to turn it alkaline, make it hard water. But it's going to involve a trek.'

It is a cruel joke that the finest beaches on St Helena lie uselessly at several hundred metres above sea level. I parked my Land Rover by the restored curtain wall up against a large military lime kiln in Sandy Bay. The kiln stands at the bottom of an old mule track, now denuded and partly torn away. The track climbs over the ridge into Potato Bay, a large uninhabited area that is a hostile shambles of raw, volcanic debris and scree slopes. After half an hour I crossed the spine of the ridge into the cupped valley head of Potato Bay, where the military quarry lay, blindingly white in the fierce midday sun: a thick deposit of coralline sand. All I needed was a deckchair and a tequila – well, and the sea.

I filled my rucksack with the silky sand and endeavoured to lift it. Too heavy. I manipulated the leaden mass onto a boulder and managed to pull it across onto my bent back, then very slowly, careful not to slip and break an ankle under the burden, I worked my way back down the ridge, doubled over into a L-shape, awkward but effective. It turned out I had scooped up thirty-three kilos of sand.

Back at Farm Lodge, Steve bailed out and cleaned the water trough, which fed into several paddocks, and I poured in fifteen kilos of this luxurious mineral, confident that the acidic water would chew away at the particles to create hard water laden with dissolved calcium.

The lambs would sup calcium every day.

Time would tell if we'd won. Meanwhile, I toiled away fanatically in the jungle of Rose Cottage, anxiously waiting for the report on my CT scan. It was like an archaeological dig. So far, I had excavated a reversible horse plough, a cannon wheel, the ornate treadle from a set of sack scales, and charming fragments of Chinese porcelain hand-painted with willow trees, sampans and trellised gardens.

Then, a small miracle. I was ferreting deep under the densely entwined branches of a thicket and dragged aside a rotting bough. A familiar angry face stared back at me. I eagerly pulled it out of the leaf mould.

It was the second foo dog.

Surely this was a good omen, to find a pair of lucky guardians for my stone gate jambs. A witty friend of mine dubbed them Foxtrot and Oscar. Well, Foxy at least, to obscure the meaning.

News back from Farm Lodge was positive. No more broken-backed lambs. The calcium drink had worked. Another zebra put to bed. But, as ever, Professor Jennings was proved right. There are plenty of zebras to go around. For all of us.

It seemed to me that my exertions with the heavy rucksack of sand had exacerbated the grotesque sensation of strangulation in my throat, and since then it had waxed and waned. But there was something else, something altogether strange: the cathedral bells of tinnitus and a mild sensation of light-headedness, which I had at first dismissed as psychosomatic, but whose reality I could no longer deny. I put it to Dr Kamar that something was interfering with my tenth cranial nerve, the vagus, otherwise known as 'the wanderer'.

Self-diagnosis is a dangerous game, but I was on the mark. Dr Kamar emailed me. My CT report was back. No mass in the pharynx, which lifted an oppressive burden. Thank you, foo dogs. But, instead, a curious observation that I had excessively elongated styloid bones, projections from the base of the skull that provide an anchor for some of the muscles involved in swallowing. And that the symptoms tentatively suggested the rarely diagnosed Eagle syndrome, where the styloids prod at a group of cranial nerves, creating the phantom, unswallowable lump – a globus – and the other extraneous symptoms. It is most prevalent in menopausal women, which I am not, age range thirty to fifty years, which I have exceeded, and those that have had a tonsillectomy, which I haven't. So, rare on rare. An outlier.

I had opened the stable door to find no common hack, but my own damned zebra. Braying heartily, no doubt, at the perfect irony.

Yet it was better news than some of the other alternatives. I had been feeling trapped. It's eight months now since I ostensibly retired, but I'm still operating and providing essential services. Until I'm replaced I have no choice, a prisoner of my ethics. My ongoing reward has been working with one of the finest, most loyal teams on the island, colleagues I can call family.

Now, though, I tackle everything with renewed vigour. Only yesterday, I went around to Plantation House and fed old Jonathan, collected faecal samples for the next phase of research in the tortoise microbiome project (tucking them in the freezer under my peas), castrated a guinea pig and remodelled a dog's knee for a luxating patella.

There's time yet to shape up my ruined Georgian pile, to clear the jungle and to bonsai my unruly, thirty-foot coffee trees into better-yielding bushes. The ultimate aim? To sit on the beautifully curved, black basalt porch steps, currently leading up into thin air, while enjoying the flavour and aroma of my own medium-roast, £600-a-kilo, green-tipped Bourbon Arabica. From half a salvaged Chinese tea bowl perhaps. That's not a bad incentive at all.

I'm grateful that my veterinary qualification has led me down an obscure, exotic path peppered with variety, surprise and delight – and the occasional browsing zebra – along with many insights into the arcane wonders of the natural world. And with, of course, Jonathan, my chelonian pal, forever lurking in the bushes; or at least for a good while yet.

And it never ends. The landline is ringing. It's the indispensable Kerry.

'I see you're coming in to do the export paperwork for Kerisha's cats?'

'Yup. Third time lucky.' Between lack of cargo space and Starsky's bladder problems we've cancelled twice already.

'Could you check a dog for me? It's got a large lump. And we've done Katy's glucose curve to adjust her insulin.'

'Yes, of course.'

'Oh, and Rosemarie said call by the Store on your way in, she's some cake for your tea.'

'Bless her!'

Animals are pure innocents, devoid of malice or deceit. They are patients that cannot speak but have many languages. They are sentient. They must not be left to suffer in silence. It is a vet's bounden duty not only to hear them but to listen to them. I have always tried to do so. I like to believe I mostly win, though sometimes, of course, I lose. Such is life.

In the end though, as my paternal grandfather taught me, it's not so much whether you win or lose but, more importantly, how you play the game.

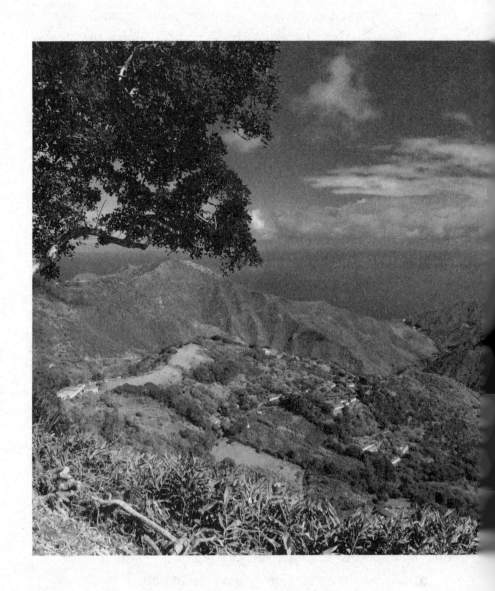

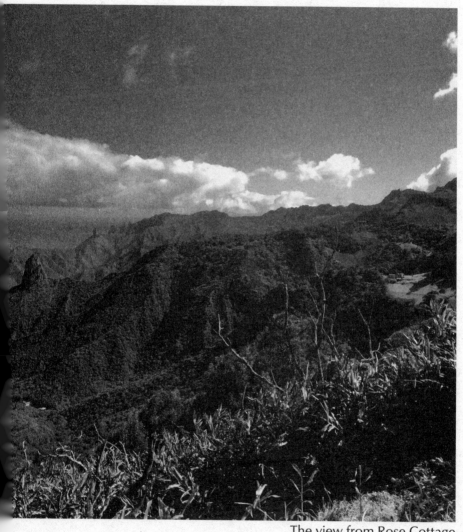

The view from Rose Cottage

ACKNOWLEDGEMENTS

Honing a manuscript into its final shape and form is the creative process not of one, but of many. I ask those I have failed to acknowledge to forgive me.

I would like to thank my agent, Annabel Merullo, of Peters, Fraser and Dunlop, for seeking me out and encouraging me to embark on this venture. I am truly indebted to the team at Duckworth Books, especially lovely Rowan Cope, my editor, for her gentle steer and for wielding her scalpel – and on occasion, machete – with surgical precision. I sent her five sheep when she only really wanted four, but she spared most of the fifth with merciful restraint. And thank you to Mia van Wyk, a fine artist in the true sense of the word, for her exquisite illustrations.

In the Falkland Islands, Steve Pointing, Phyl Rendell and Sue Harvey set me on a rewarding island path, and Sarah Bowles buoyed me up with her crisp humour, invaluable skills, and succulent mutton roasts. Paul Brickle, toothfish guru and fisheries supremo, inspired me with his enthusiasm for all things briny.

On St Helena my work would have been overwhelming were it not for the loyalty of my superb team: Ken 'Harp' Henry, Kerry Sim, Rico 'Turby' Williams, and Clayton 'Chopsie' Andrews. I never heard a surly word, was never refused assistance at ungodly hours, and humour and positivity prevailed even in the direst of moments. Thanks also to my line manager, Andrea

Timm, for her approachability and wholehearted support, and the man at the helm, Darren Duncan, for his friendship and quietly spoken wisdom. Governors Mark Capes, Andrew Gurr and Philip Rushbrook each took on the unexpected role of tortoise caretaker, assisted me with Jonathan's care and extended their hospitality to me on many occasions.

The islanders of Tristan da Cunha enfolded me into their tightly knit community, a privilege and an indelible bond I shall carry to the grave. Specifically, I would like to thank the Island Council. They listened, analysed then pronounced their rulings with steadfast logic and unimpeachable clarity.

And finally, there are those who have gone before us and are an integral part of these stories: the charismatic Lewis Glass, the drily laconic Leon Berntsen, the illustrious Captain Rodney Young, and genial Sean Burns, Administrator of Tristan, who enabled and facilitated several of my initiatives. We miss you, but you live on in our memories.